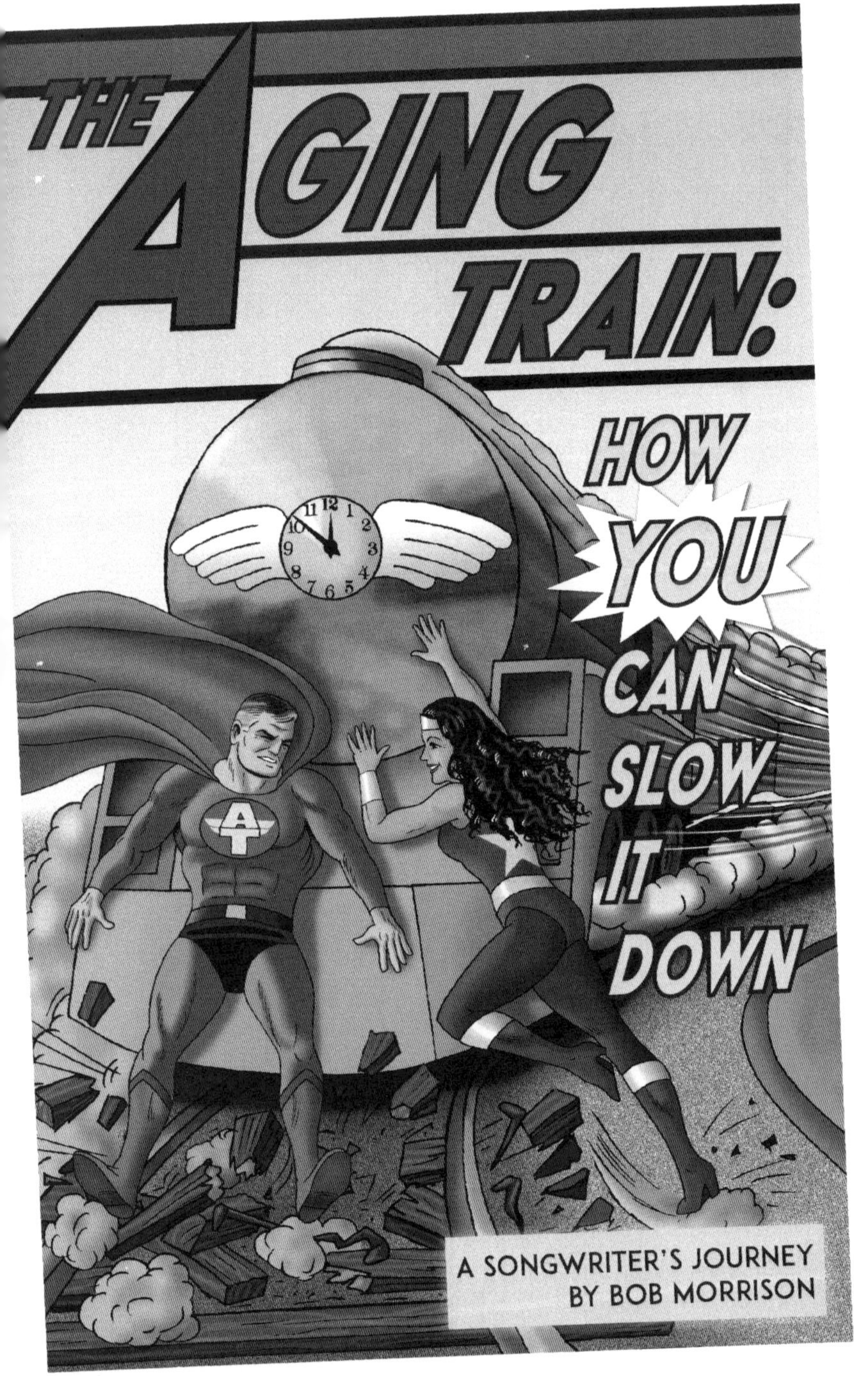
THE AGING TRAIN:
HOW YOU CAN SLOW IT DOWN
A SONGWRITER'S JOURNEY
BY BOB MORRISON

Published by McClearen Creative
Nashville, Tennessee
www.mcclearencreative.com

Art Direction, Design & Illustrations by McClearen Creative:
Design by Brenda McClearen
Illustrations by Randy Garrett

Photography by Bev Moser

Identifiers: LCCN 2019956964 (print) | ISBN-978-1-7329228-1-5 (paperback)
Printed in the United States of America

DEDICATION

To my daughters, Wendy and Andrea, who,
though taking different paths in life,
became true inspirations to me.

From the Author —
A Disclaimer Of Sorts

When I started writing this material four years ago, I simply intended a diary of my experiences. I never entertained the notion that it would become a book, much less be published. It was just something fun to do. Most of my comments and opinions on these pages have been researched, but I didn't know that a non-fiction book can only have credibility if the sources are meticulously researched and cataloged. Because of my lack of knowledge, I didn't record the sources at the time. When I learned that it was a necessity, and tried to go back to recreate the list, I discovered some of the source material was impossible to find, appearing in magazines rather than on the internet. This being the case, I believe each reader needs to explore and depend on their own experiences, suspicions, and convictions. Even with the constant bombardment of mis- and disinformation, we all have strong inclinations of where the truth most likely is. But there are those whose job it is to manipulate and distort the facts. They know exactly how to confuse the issue and cover their tracks. Bad intentions and malfeasance are hard to prove. The good news is that I recovered many of the sources and found new sources for some of the material.

Since proving what I say is beyond the scope of this book, my readers would do well to depend on their own research and gut, as I always have and will continue to do. Someone once said everything is a scam to a greater or lesser extent. Bottom line? You have the right to take everything I say in this book with a grain of salt. Decide the merits or lack thereof for yourself.

Acknowledgements

The personal workout program I'd been doing was working so well for me, I thought there might be others who could reap some of the same benefits I was enjoying. Unfortunately, I knew absolutely nothing about what was required to organize and write a book. It's a totally different animal than songwriting. I was completely lost, but I had some friends who gave me feedback and direction that led me to think that maybe there was a book there. I'd like to thank all those who helped in small and larger ways.

My first reader was Carolyn Sells. She is a no-nonsense, longtime friend who for years worked at Combine Music, my legendary song publisher. She was a secretary, but she was much more than that. Thank you, C., for your consistent candor and encouragement.

Then came the second reader, Gynny Butler, my wife's cousin from New York. She was a native New Yorker who moved to Nashville after the 9-11 happened. Krissi, her daughter, and Dave, her son, also read the rough draft and gave some valuable insights. Thanks to each.

Kerry O'Neil, one of the true movers and shakers on Music Row in Nashville, and I have been business associates and friends for some forty years. He was my accountant in the early days and eventually branched out very successfully into music publishing and other entrepreneurial endeavors. I could always depend on him for a straight answer, whether positive or negative. I was aware that he'd written books and gone through the process. Thanks, K., for your suggestions and for the names of people I should contact to get to the next step.

My first editor was Cathy Kodra, a published poet. She was my first teacher, my first exposure to reality. She helped me go from being lost to at least understanding what I needed to do to make a diary into something that would resemble a book. Cathy, I appreciate your skill and your patience. This wouldn't have happened without you. A big thanks.

The look of the book was the work of Brenda McClearen of McClearen Creative. The cover design, layout, and all the exercise illustrations were contributions of her company. To explain an exercise is not easy. But the images were worth a thousand words. It was great. I didn't have to write as many descriptions. But that was only part of what she did. At my urging, she jumped in and helped me with every aspect of making "The Aging Train" a better book. She knew what the book was lacking and helped me get where it needed to go. I went from liking the book to being proud of it.

Thanks, Brenda McC

A Beta reader is someone who reads the edited text and finds areas that are unclear and should be better explained. They also make suggestions about the organization, readability, and interest in

the book. My choices were Doug Bennett, one of my long-time best friends and golf buddy, and Wendy Morrison, my daughter, who majored in English at Sewanee and taught it for many years at the Asheville School in Asheville, N.C. Doug was basics, nuts and bolts, then Wendy was the more organizational and technical side. I needed what both offered and it couldn't have worked out better. They both did a wonderful job of pointing out flaws, some small, some large, and improving what was there.
My thanks to you both.

TABLE OF CONTENTS

The Aging Train: How _You_ Can Slow It Down

······

**Without deviation from the norm,
progress is not possible.
—Frank Zappa**

······

Preface

Aging is like being a passenger on a runaway train. If we do nothing but sit and ride, the train will start to pick up speed, and continue to go downhill until the day we reach our final destination. So far, no one I know has been able to figure out a way to get off the train, but I do believe in many cases, the aging process can be slowed down. Of course, it can also be sped up. I believe there is another, better way than hoping for the best. Not everything in individual wellness can be controlled. We're all born with inherent health weaknesses, strengths, and vulnerabilities which can be enabled or suppressed to some extent by the choices we make. That's what this book is about.

There is an old saying: "You can't teach an old dog new tricks." Well, that depends on the old dog. When I turned seventy, I decided to make some changes to my workout schedule and my health regimen. Though I had exercised nearly all my adult life and was by all criteria doing well for my age, I wanted to try something else, a different road. I felt that I might be spending more time than necessary to get the results I wanted. My question was: Could I work out less and get anywhere near the benefits of what I for so long had been doing? At that time, writing a book wasn't on the radar. I never once thought about it until I realized what was happening—I was getting everything I'd hoped for and more! Less time, better results, no exhaustion. I've been told I don't look my age, I've gotten stronger, and, just maybe, I might live longer than my genetic makeup and national statistics would predict. I began to see that by making some different choices, it might be possible to slow down the aging train everyone is on.

Our culture almost demands that we be in a hurry. The reasons are varied and complicated. Lives are busier than ever. Kids are being shuttled everywhere, with both parents working to make ends meet. Instead of saving us time, technology seems to be stealing time, leaving less for real communication with those who matter most. It occurred to me that maybe others could benefit from my experience.

With the research that was involved in the writing process, I began to think a lot about fingerprints. The whorls and swirls at the tips of our fingers. We've always heard that fingerprints are one of a kind. Unique. Even identical twins don't have the same fingerprints. There are 7.4 billion people on the earth at present, give or take a few hundred thousand. Everyone with a different fingerprint. That's what we've always heard. The same thing is said about snowflakes—water that has frozen into an infinite number of crystalline forms. It would be hard to prove or disprove these common beliefs, but it brings up a fascinating point. Suppose we apply the differences that occur with individual fingerprints to the complexity of the individual human body?

It's not hard to assume from the examples above that nature doesn't deal in duplicates. And if so, rarely. Everything in nature, despite obvious similarities, is very possibly one of a kind. What about each of us? We appear to be a random arrangement of infinite combinations. A crazy blob of protoplasm, flesh, and blood with no particular rhyme or reason to the combinations. Geniuses are born of parents with average intelligence; dullards are born of brilliant parents. We all think, feel, and respond differently to practically everything. Siblings can be polar opposites in personality, political beliefs, food preferences and in many other ways. Differences also mean differences in our individual chemistry. There are similarities, of course, in how we behave, but we are not identical. I believe this is why the medical profession is often a hit-or-miss proposition. The same drug will cure one person and kill another, sometimes in the same family. Though Mother Nature is often a fickle mistress, I feel she is more reliable than man. There's no profit motive in nature.

Several years ago, I read something Isaac Azimov once said in an interview that resonated with me. This prolific writer (five hundred books, including many works of science fiction), made the comment, "Ninety percent of all science fiction is crap." He hesitated a moment and then said, "As a matter of fact, ninety percent of everything is crap." This became one of my mantras. An Oprah "Aha moment." What a simple yet profound way to look at the world! I don't know whether the percentages are accurate, but he stumbled upon something I never thought about it until I read an excerpt from the interview. It applies to art, talking heads, politicians, and people in general—just about anything you look at closely. A good way to approach this world might be with the intent of finding that elusive ten percent. The better and the best of us. The other ninety percent of humanity is made up of those individuals who don't qualify to a greater or lesser extent. For me, the top ten percent would be the ones with, in varying degrees, talent, a sense of humor about the world and themselves, intelligence, social responsibility, and a lack of arrogance. Good-hearted and honest people, good friends, good caring doctors, good plumbers, the good of everything. We don't seem to have an overabundance of them.

Because of Azimov, I look for the ten percent. I don't always find them, but I always keep looking. In the pages that follow, I'll mention the ten percent rule again. I just wanted to share this little story first.

About the Author

I was born in 1942 in Biloxi, Mississippi. I was a teenager when the rock and roll era in music began. Remember jukeboxes? That was my dad's business. He would put a jukebox in a hotel bar, honky-tonk or restaurant, keep it in working order, add five new records every two weeks to keep the music current. He would bring me a set of all the new records, and though I didn't realize it at the time, I was getting a free commercial music education. I was exposed at an early age to rhythm and blues, country, and "pop" (which in those days meant Frank Sinatra and Tony Bennett—amazingly, he is still performing at 93!) and of course, the new raucous arrival on the musical block, "Rock and Roll," which at that time, was labeled the "devil's music" by some in religious organizations. What began as an interest in music soon turned into a passion for me. I started listening to the radio for new songs and giving my dad suggestions on what I thought might be a hit. I didn't know what I didn't know, but I got a strange shivery feeling somewhere between my heart and gut when I heard a new record that somehow did something to me. At fifteen, for Christmas, I received my first guitar, a real inexpensive one from Sears, finally got it in tune, and after a few years of practice, started "sitting in" with a local rock band.

After high school, I went to Mississippi State University on a track scholarship where I performed and started writing songs. I graduated with a degree in nuclear engineering and, illogically, decided to enter the music business. I sang in clubs on the East Coast and signed with Columbia Records in New York. Later I moved to Hollywood and signed with Screen-Gems TV as a contract actor. I subsequently left Columbia Records and signed with Capitol Records where I recorded and released a self-penned album, *Friends of Mine*.

In 1973 I moved to Nashville, signed with Combine Music, one of Music Row's top independent publishers, and had my first success as a writer with a song called *"The River's Too Wide"* which was recorded by Olivia Newton-John. Over the next several years, I co-wrote *"Angels, Roses, and Rain,"* a number one record for Dickey Lee; *"Midnight Angel"* by Barbara Mandrell; Reba McEntire's first top-ten record, *"Up To Heaven"*; and the Oak Ridge Boys' hit, *"You're the One (In a Million),"* which was later used by the ABC television network as its national promo song.

In 1978 I was named the ASCAP (The American Society of Composers Authors and Publishers) Country Songwriter of the Year. In 1979 I won a Grammy for *"You Decorated My Life,"* co-written with Debbie Hupp, and in 1980, I received two Grammy nominations: Best country song (*"Lookin' For Love"*) and Best Album Written for a Motion Picture (Urban Cowboy). I won another ASCAP Songwriter of the Year in 1980, and again in 1981 and 1982. I was voted NSAI (Nashville Songwriters Association

International) Writer of the Year in 1980. Altogether I won forty-six ASCAP awards. In 2006, I was nominated for the Nashville Songwriter's Hall of Fame. In 2016, I was inducted.

Included among over two hundred recordings of my songs are:

Lookin' For Love — Johnny Lee

You Decorated My Life — Kenny Rogers

You're the One (In a Million) — The Oak Ridge Boys

Tonight, the Heartache's on Me — The Dixie Chicks

Whiskey, If You Were a Woman — Highway 101

Love the World Away — Kenny Rogers (from Urban Cowboy)

Shine On — George Jones

Born to Love Me — Ray Charles

Don't Call Him a Cowboy — Conway Twitty

I Still Believe in Waltzes — Conway Twitty & Loretta Lynn

You'd Make an Angel Wanna Cheat — The Kendalls

All My Roads — Ronnie Milsap

The Grandest Lady of Them All — Conway Twitty

Up to Heaven — Reba McEntire

Make-Believe It's Your First Time — The Carpenters

The River's Too Wide — Olivia Newton-John

Let Me Be Your Baby — Charly McClain

A songwriter—or any creative person for that matter—is at risk for a short shelf life. Such was the case with me and many of my peers. The reasons are complex and have as much to do with the individual artist or writer as with the constant changing of the guard. It's a youth-oriented business, as many are, and growing older is not an advantage.

An independent songwriter has little power, even during his successful years. "No" is so easy for music execs to say. There are many reasons why they say no—some reasons fall under the heading of "hidden agendas." It might be where they are emotionally that morning. Good luck playing a love song to a music exec with a hangover who just had a big fight with his significant other. There are also business reasons. If they don't have a financial stake in songs you are playing for them, they are less inclined to record your song over one they do have an interest in. And once career momentum is lost, that's pretty much it. Fortunately, I didn't buy twelve Cadillacs or acquire four wives, and I had a very conservative approach to finances. I didn't spend it, I invested it. I knew the day would come when I wouldn't matter, my fifteen minutes of fame would be over. Truth? If it weren't for a couple of copyrights I happened to have been a part of, I have no idea what I would be doing today. But I'm reasonably sure I wouldn't be living the life I'm living now.

As time passed and my songwriting career faded in the rearview mirror, I grew more and more curious. I wanted to know things. I wanted to know the why. I had learned a lot, but could never figure out why we are here. I concluded that since I didn't have a clue, and didn't know whether I'd make another appearance on earth in another life sometime in the future, I might as well do the best I can with whatever modest gifts I have now.

About the Photos

Spoiler alert:
I don't look like a young
   Arnold Schwarzenegger.

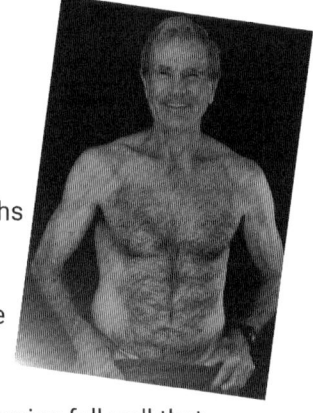

   I decided to have these photographs
taken when I was about to turn
seventy-five. Why? You might think
it's an exercise in vanity, and you have
a right to that opinion. The truth is, I
wanted to make a permanent visual
record of where I was at this time, knowing full well that
this might be the best it's going to get for me. I started
this whole process with one goal in mind: to get in the
best shape possible for my age. That's it. I thought that
was the best road to better health and vitality. How I look
physically was an unintended but positive consequence
of the process. I've never had anything close to a six-
pack, even when I was in top shape in college days on
the track team. The reason is, no matter how many ab
exercises you do, you have to get rid of the fat covering
them; otherwise, they will stay hidden.

   The photos were taken by Bev Moser, one of the
more talented photographers in Nashville. She had taken
some photos of me for NSAI for the Hall of Fame cer-
emony. I told her I was going to come out to her studio
and take some topless photos when I got up the nerve,
but she laughed, thinking I was pulling her leg. These are
the result. They haven't been photoshopped or altered.

••••••

Note: All noncredited quotes in this book belong to the author.

25

The Aging Train: How _You_ Can Slow It Down

CHAPTER 1
Introduction—What I've Learned

I have always had a workout regimen except for one brief period after college when I gained twenty pounds, reaching 180, my highest weight before or since. After a lot of years, I learned that high-intensity, anaerobic workouts have a lot of advantages over aerobic workouts though both have health benefits. (Aerobic means working out and keeping up with your oxygen needs. Anaerobic is a more intense workout where for a time you can't keep up with your oxygen needs.) Anaerobic is less time consuming, has more fat-burning potential, and it builds a surprising amount of endurance without long boring workouts in freezing or blistering weather. It's pretty amazing. The secret is that anaerobic exercise releases human growth hormone (HGH) in the body naturally, which apparently slows down the aging process. The downside? You have to get into shape before you can do the workout, and reaching that point is not easy. It takes six months or so, and maybe even longer.

Many celebrities, athletes, and entertainers receive HGH injections. This method appears to have some of the same benefits of exercise, but also some downsides. I'd much rather do the work and have nature produce the results than pay a hefty sum for an outside agent. I've always believed more in Mother Nature than in the sometimes questionable nature of medical technology. I'm not afraid of needles, but I try to avoid man-made injections whenever possible.

Factoring in my age, I'm now in better shape overall than at any time in my life. Before this work-out regimen, I was 6'1' and weighed 163, a weight I stayed at for many years (with the exception of the time between Thanksgiving and Christmas when I usually gain a few extra pounds). I now weigh 152 pounds. Don't think I've lost any height, but I haven't checked.

······

**"Finishing first is not always best...
take life, for example."
—Van Kussrow III**

**"Moderation in everything.
Including moderation."
—Sheila Meadows,
Nashville chiropractor**

······

CHAPTER 2
Following Your Yellow Brick Road: Where Are You Now and Where Do You Want to Be?

If you're reading this, you are perhaps interested in changing direction in your life. You may be healthy for "your age" but need a few outside-the-box ideas to help you get better for your age. You may just be curious. If you're looking for an easy way to the promised land, this might not be the right book for you. What is contained within is hard, or I should say, as hard as you want to make it. But you will get something back for the work you do. Always.

Changes are not easy to make. We humans are creatures of habit, and we love our rituals. We often go through life with very little thought. My morning rituals are so ingrained that an outsider probably couldn't tell the difference from one day to the next. Routines set up over a long period of time usually end up in what we call our comfort zone. Unfortunately, habits and the resulting comfort zone lead some of us into an unhealthy, uncomfortable place. If you're in a good place and you're happy with how you feel and look, that's great. If not, then maybe some changes—even just small ones—need to be made. We all love the familiarity of our chosen Yellow Brick Road. We know where it leads. We can walk it in our sleep. But if you're interested in reinventing yourself, you have to fight inertia, the tendency for a body at rest to remain at rest. I'm not only talking about physical rest, such as napping. I'm also talking about mental rest. The greatest obstacle to anything we do is our own mind. The easiest thing to do in life is to say no. The next easiest thing to do is nothing.

Research tells us we only use a small part of our brains. I think that applies to our physical bodies as well. Many people have successfully reinvented themselves. They were willing to try different things, full well knowing they could fail. The defunct television show *"The Biggest Losers"* is one example. I know it's a cliché, but I believe there is no such thing as failing if you try. No one can move forward by choosing to stay in the same place. Or by keeping the same habits and routines. Something has to change, or else nothing will.

The Backstory

My paternal grandfather, Buck, died at fifty years of age. I never knew him. My mother was pregnant with me at the time. Buck's earthly departure might have been hastened by being married to a brittle and difficult woman, my paternal grandmother, Juanita (I called her Maump). I spent enough time around her to know she was no June Cleaver, or such was my youthful perception. One of the truly amusing things my grandmother said when she was in her seventies, which I remember to this day, was, "I don't mind dying. I just don't want to stop breathing first."

The women in both my parents' families lived to their middle to later eighties. My grandmother on my dad's side was cogent and sharp until the end. My mother's family was a study in poverty and contradiction. Ed Marshall, my maternal grandfather, was twenty-eight when he married Mae, sixteen. They had seven children. Two were boys: Charles, when young, a pretty good boxer and later a fisherman; and George, a career military man (with anger issues—he was busted in rank three times, I believe) who could sing pretty well, Irish tenor-like. The five girls were Eva, Vera, Helen, Violet, and my mom Myrtis, the youngest.

Grandpa Ed once worked for the railroad and was either let go or retired. My grandmother Mae birthed and raised the seven children, operated a boarding house, and planted and worked a large vegetable garden. She washed clothes in the old rub board way and hung them on the line. She cooked for her large family and even made meals for her boarders. I don't know how she did it. She was the hardest working woman I have ever seen. She lived a long life, well into her eighties with her faculties intact. She would have been a good grandmother if she'd had the time. I'm not complaining. I'd never experienced a "normal" grandchild/grandparent relationship, so I didn't see anything amiss. What you don't know is sometimes a good thing. Given

31

the individuals involved, maybe it was a good thing. My parents were loving, and I never felt there was anything unusual or missing in not having a grand-parent relationship.

Mom's parents lived in the house next to us before I was born, so as I grew up, I got a firsthand childhood view of her family. Ed, who we called "Dad," was kind of a cantankerous deadbeat. A stoop-shouldered, unshaven old coot, he was also foul-mouthed and lazy. He had two drooling, stinking bulldogs, which he kept in the house. My mother hated those dogs. As a consequence, she never allowed an animal in her house. In many years as a boy, I never saw Ed help Mae, who we called "Nan-ny." Maybe he did, but I never witnessed it. Ed called me "boy." That was it. I'm not sure he knew my name or cared.

My mother quit school when she was twelve years old. She had two reasons. Back then parents had to buy school books for their children. What little money there was in the Marshall household had to be spent on necessities. My mother was forced to sit with other kids who had books, and it was embar-rassing for her. The family also needed her to work. At twelve years old, she went to work as a waitress. Her teacher pleaded with her to stay in school because she was a very good student, but it wasn't to be. (Her teacher, Miss Priscilla Rich, became my teacher, still at Gorenflo Elementary twenty-plus years later. She asked me if I was going to be a smart as my mother. I said I didn't know.)

In 1937 my mom married my dad, Charles Morrison. She was seventeen and he was twenty-one. He had graduated from Biloxi High School. He'd been raised Catholic, she Lutheran. They agreed not to have children for five years to make sure their marriage stayed on solid ground. I was their first child, and their last. My mom had a miscarriage several years later and was not able to have more children. But they made it work. My parents let me have a long leash. Curious about what words were and what they meant, I learned to read before I entered first grade. My dad was a jukebox operator, a business he co-owned with his brother George, and my mom was a housewife. They supported me in everything I did. I played Little League baseball at nine years old, Babe Ruth League, and high school baseball, basketball, and track. I had a brief flirtation with football in junior high, but with my 115-pound ectomorphic body, it was sanctioned suicide. I quickly came to my senses and left the sport to those who outweighed me by forty to seventy pounds. I had a sport for all seasons, so it wasn't a great loss. Some of my favorite memories are of Mom, Dad, and I piling into the car and traveling to baseball and basketball games and track meets. My parents were there for every single one.

Three events helped shape my attitude and decisions regarding the health profession in general and my personal vulnerability, specifically. One was the death of my father, the victim of a medical mistake. When he was fifty-three, he had an intestinal blockage and needed an operation to clear the obstruction. He had to have a second operation for I don't know what reason. They took his intestines out and washed them in a saline solution. He later died of something called peritonitis. I was twenty-seven and didn't know exactly what that was. Later on, **M.A.S.H.**, a TV series about a mobile army surgical hospital in the Korean War, an arrogant colonel operated on a wounded soldier who, when he should have been getting better, kept getting progressively worse. Hawkeye (Alan Alda), a more competent surgeon, diagnosed peritonitis, which meant that bowel contents were leaking into the abdominal cavity. Hawkeye redid the surgery, and the soldier started improving immediately. Otherwise, he would have lapsed into sepsis and died. Hollywood ending: hero triumphs. No such luck for my dad. A stitch might have been missed somehow in the sewing-up process. Before the operation, I tried to talk my dad into going to Ochsner Clinic in New Orleans. He said his surgeon would be fine. We later found out the surgeon was an alcoholic, though there may have been no connection with what happened.

Then there was watching my mom's mind slowly being taken away by Alzheimer's. As it turned out, all of my mom's siblings ended up with this dreaded disease. All seven died from its complications. My family history suggested that longevity for me would be iffy at best. I found myself staring down a double-barreled shotgun. I asked myself what would happen if I became my own experiment. If I did things differently, could that help me beat the odds? I didn't know where to start or what things to do, but in true American fashion, I took a leap of faith. What did I have to lose? It would have to be a learning by doing—and perhaps failing—thing.

The coup de grace was the death of my younger daughter in 2010 at age thirty-seven. In a misdiagnosis, the doctor concluded she had some form of IBS. I was worried because she had been a great swimmer at the University of Georgia and she just wasn't responding to the treatment being offered. Though she had always stayed fit, she now had very little energy. On the Friday before she passed away, I asked her doctor to see her, and he declined. She died that Sunday. An autopsy suggested she had died from the complications of lupus. We were out of town. Not only was this a tragic and infuriating ending for us, but it also affected a lot of people. The loss was not only ours but the community's as well. She was a wonderful counselor at Eakin Elementary—K through 4—in Nashville, serving a large percentage of inner-city students. Earlier that year she'd been runner-up for teacher of the year in Davidson County. At her visitation, eight hundred people came to say goodbye. She still resonates in the hallways of the Eakin school. The final blow came when my wife and I and Andrea's widower husband made an appointment with her doctor to talk to him about the situation. He chose not to show up. With regard to this whole episode, a songwriter friend who had also experienced the death of a child said to me, "You never get over it, but you can sometimes get around it."

The lesson I took away from the loss of my father and my daughter was: Don't trust someone just because he or she has a medical degree. Do your homework. Make sure you have the best man or woman for the job, and realize that even the best make mistakes. Am I prejudiced against the medical profession? Somewhat, because of personal experiences. But I'd like to believe I'm more wary and pragmatic than prejudicial. My mom used to feel that doctors were somehow specially anointed individuals with almost magical superhuman powers. Some might be, but I don't feel that. We all have the unfortunate characteristic of being human, where imperfection is there in varying degrees and sometimes runs rampant. I've been lucky to find truly good ones for the most part. When I occasionally find someone my gut tells me to be wary of, I bid them sayonara and look elsewhere. My gut has been right more times than not. So far. It could be that I've just been lucky.

So back to that shotgun. In many ways, I had a distinct advantage over my forebears. Both my grandfather and father smoked cigarettes. A lot of cigarettes. I remember my dad smoking two packs of Pall Malls a day. Every day. In their respective generations, smoking was the norm. There was nothing to fear as far as the public was concerned, and everybody did it— think **Mad Men**, the critically acclaimed AMC show about the fifties. The insidious nature of the habit was not well known back then except by top executives of the tobacco industry who didn't feel it necessary to let anyone else know.

Fortunately, I never smoked. And unlike my father and grandfather, I was an athlete of sorts who naïvely believed as a teenager that my sports heroes, like Jack Armstrong the All-American boy, would always treat our fairer sex like ladies, bathe frequently, and never smoke. There was a rumor floating around that cigarettes didn't improve athletic performance, so I resisted the temptation to be cool, which I wouldn't have known how to be anyway. I dealt with the peer pressure and even put aside my admiration for Humphrey Bogart, who smoked a lot in films— and who died at fifty-seven—and never started down that road. I never knew I was being smart. Sometimes it's great to be naïve.

••••••

"Genetics is the gun, but lifestyle pulls the trigger."
—Brooke Kalanick, N.D.
(Naturopathic Physician)

••••••

Why Play Russian Roulette?

In the May/June 2011 issue of Natural Health magazine, I came across an interesting article stating that thirty to forty percent of an individual's health is determined by genetics, and sixty to seventy percent can be attributed to lifestyle. The percentages are probably dependent on the individual. Some might have a higher genetic tendency, some lower. According to the writer, what we eat, how and how much we exercise, and the way we deal with stress all have a say. If this premise is true and people with a family history of cancer follows the same life habits as their parents did, it may be that they're leaving the door ajar to the same problems. The article implied that you might be able to dodge the family bullet by altering your lifestyle. Well, I'm a believer that nothing is etched in stone, and that everything we do has consequences, positive or negative. Why not hedge the bet? Seems to me we have nothing to lose.

FYI: Recently **60 Minutes** had a report on CRISPR, a genetic editing tool that promises to be a game changer. It can take the flaws in individual DNA and fix them, much as you might correct spelling in this paragraph. The scientists believe it can eradicate certain diseases by repairing the responsible gene. The science is in its infancy, but stay tuned. It could happen.

CHAPTER 3
The Big Questions

What do we know for sure?

If nothing else, I'm outspoken. Too much so, if you ask my wife of fifty years. Truth? I only know truth from my perspective. You have to decide what is true for you. I've lived over seventy years and in time realized that our health is our responsibility. No one else's. There are people who can help and information that can help, but ultimately the ball is in our court.

We know for sure we can't always depend on doctors. It would be interesting to know the statistics of every disastrously wrong diagnosis that has led to serious problems, even death. I believe that these numbers are known but not published, and that more than a few doctors move around a lot because of an abnormally high rate of poor outcomes or patient deaths.

But to be fair, I have to say there are many great people in the health care system—conscientious, caring, and skilled. It's a very stressful, and at times, difficult profession. Each doctor, nurse, and staff member holds someone's life in their hands. Unfortunately, mistakes, whether negligent or innocent, can be fatal. I have had more than my share of really skilled doctors, nurses, and good health care outcomes throughout my life. There have also been a few disastrous outcomes with those I love. But I want to make sure to give credit to the many qualified and good people out there. It's up to us to find them.

FYI—In 2009 The World Health Organization (WHO) did a study of the health costs and actual results of every country that had a health system. Statistically, the U.S. was #1 in costs—by far— and #37 in outcomes. Here's their list.[1]

1.	France	21.	Belgium
2.	Italy	22.	Colombia
3.	San Marino	23.	Sweden
4.	Andorra	24.	Cyprus
5.	Malta	25.	Germany
6.	Singapore	26.	Saudi Arabia
7.	Spain	27.	United Arab Emirates
8.	Oman	28.	Israel
9.	Austria	29.	Morocco
10.	Japan	30.	Canada
11.	Norway	31.	Finland
12.	Portugal	32.	Australia
13.	Monaco	33.	Chile
14.	Greece	34.	Denmark
15.	Iceland	35.	Dominica
16.	Luxembourg	36.	Costa Rica
17.	Netherlands	37.	USA***
18.	United Kingdom		
19.	Ireland		
20.	Switzerland		

The above notwithstanding, we know that the cost of care and medication continues to rise. A long article in *Time* magazine (2013)[2], titled "Bitter Pill," chronicled the egregious pricing in the hospital business. It appears that the malfeasance and bad judgment, in general, is top-down. I always snarkily say, "Guess the CEO really needs another house to go with his other three." If you think this is unfair, you should look up some of their yearly salaries. Moreover, non-profit hospitals don't exist, according to the article. Creative bookkeeping can prove anything, and the markups on medical devices and drugs are scandalous.

Big Pharma is just one more example of corporations that seem to lack evidence of social responsibility. Their number one job is selling us pills. And they're good at it. We know the U.S. pays significantly more than other countries for its top prescription drugs.[3] We know medications always involve risks, and our health problems must be assessed as worth those risks. There are many instances when people do need medication, and some are life-and-death matters, but I believe many prescribed drugs could be reduced or eliminated with appropriate lifestyle changes.

Recently, the pharmaceutical industry has come under increasing scrutiny, mostly because of the opioid crisis. And that's not the only troubling fact. According to *US News and World Report* (2016), over one hundred thousand of our citizens die every year due to the side effects of doctor-prescribed drugs taken as directed.[4]

As if we need any more evidence to question the questionable practices of most of the pharmaceutical companies and medical device manufacturers, the FDA recently reported brand-name drug makers were refusing to let generic drug makers buy the samples necessary to reproduce the formulas for a generic version. The reason is obvious. To keep their monopolies intact, they put off or avoid competition. By delaying generic versions, they can continue to charge exorbitant prices for necessary drugs, costing Medicare and Medicaid over ten billion dollars in 2016.[5] It's no wonder that America can't afford health care. The prices continue to go up for no clear reason except profit. Apparently, anything deemed "too big to fail" is basically untouchable.

But there are real world human consequences of the "money first" choices Big Pharma makes: the all-too-frequent stories of people having to ration or skip doses of insulin or other necessary medications because they can't afford them. Though Big Pharma likes to claim they are in the health care business, it seems they are far less in health care than in business.

As of this writing, only two countries can advertise prescription drugs on television: New Zealand and the USA.[6] To me, the countries that don't allow it make dollars and sense. Advertising costs millions, and we all know who pays for it.

We know that many of our health problems are caused by the conveniences that have crept into and become a part of our culture in the last fifty years. Food manipulation and production combined with sedentary lifestyles are a double-edged sword poised and ready to fall on those of us who don't take our health into our own hands. Living forever is not one of our options. But life can be better if we don't buy into the propaganda that makes us depend on those who don't have our best interests at heart.

What can we do?

There are myriad personality types in this world. I'm mainly interested in two broad-based types: the ones who simply let things happen and the ones who try to make things happen. True, there are a lot of events we cannot control. But there are some we can control or at least influence, negatively or positively. T.S. Eliot once said, "If you haven't the strength to impose your own terms upon life, then you must accept the terms it offers you."

The tendency toward good health is definitely related to individual DNA. Some people are born beautiful, some intelligent, and some win the sperm-and-egg lottery and are born rich. And some, through no apparent effort of their own, win the health lottery. They smoke and/or drink to excess, eat anything, never exercise, and still live a long and relatively healthy life. We all know people like this. Good for them. But some people are not so lucky. They don't win the lottery, and are destined to be ill and die relatively young. Cancer or another serious illness may be in their genetic cards. There may be a way to sidetrack or stop it, though some would strongly disagree. If you are vulnerable to certain illnesses, they can definitely be enabled. Most of us fit somewhere in between on the health spectrum—people with weaknesses but who can positively affect their health by how they live and the choices they make. It's unwise to depend on any lottery especially one that determines health.

······

Life will find your weaknesses and exploit them.

"Everybody has a good plan until the first punch lands in your face."
— Mike Tyson

"Life is short. Shorter for some than others." Gus in Lonesome Dove
— Larry McMurtry

······

Man has an unwritten covenant with nature. If we take care of nature, it takes care of us. It has provided for us for thousands of years. The human animal has adapted to changing circumstances and is amazingly flexible, chemically, mentally and physically. But one of the downfalls of man is arrogance—and greed. Both. We have this crazy, mistaken idea that we can better nature or control it to our purposes and beat it at its own game. I haven't found much evidence, outside of eliminating some deadly diseases, to support this. Every now and then man stumbles on something good that actually works. More on this later.

What do we have in common and what sets us apart?

No matter who we are and what we believe, there is one thing we have in common, one truth that is indisputable—we are not going to live forever. That is a cosmic reality in which we have no vote or voice. Herb Silverman, in his book *"Atheist Stranger in a Strange Religious Land"* wrote, "Life is a sexually transmitted disease with a 100% mortality rate." That about says it. We do have, however, as a living breathing organism—the freedom of choice. There are good choices and bad ones and they have everything to do with the speed of aging and even how soon we will die.

One thing I believe needs to be pointed out before we go forward. Though we are all of the same human species and have many characteristics in common, we also have great differences. And they are not so easily seen or known. To give you an example, a few of you may remember the world-class American long-distance runner, Jim Ryun. He would probably have won the 1500-meter run (the metric mile) in the Munich Olympics in 1972 had he not been stepped on, falling to the track, putting him too far behind to catch up. Ryun's resting heart rate was seventy. This is unusually high for a world-class athlete. Bjorn Borg, for example, the great Swedish tennis player, had a resting heart rate of thirty-five. Unusually low, but not for a world-class, trained athlete. How can two great athletes have such different numbers? It has to do with the concept of "normal." What is normal for you might not be for me. And in reality, there is no "normal." To the naked eye, we look much the same. But we have different fingerprints, different strengths and weaknesses. It's all about personal chemistry.

Do You Have to Be an Athlete to Be Healthy?

No, but if you've never been an athlete, you're at a slight disadvantage. And not for the reason you might think. Any would-be athlete, whether talented or not, whether in junior high, high school, college, or the professional ranks, has had to deal with the rigors of getting in condition and following a regimen from a coach who's the one calling the shots. Pain is part of the process. You have to learn to deal with it, and it's the only way to get the best from yourself. I saw a sign in the YMCA the other day that said, If you don't challenge yourself, nothing will change. Nobody likes to hurt, but it takes some mental toughness if you want to achieve your goals—particularly lofty ones like losing fifty pounds or running a 10K. This work is a high mental hurdle even before it becomes a physical hurdle. The challenge is, you have to make a plan and then follow through. Some of us get the best results going it alone. Others of us find success with the support of a personal trainer or an accountability partner. But ultimately, we're the adults in the room. There's no drill sergeant yelling that we are worthless, etc., to "motivate" us. The ball is in our court, and we have only ourselves to answer to. The beauty of this process is that when you persist and ignore all the voices in your head telling you "this is stupid" and "you should quit," you will surprise yourself. Once people realize what it takes and start to do the work, it gets easier. And the rewards are more self-confidence, better health, a brighter outlook, and, oddly, more energy. Much more.

Is there a point that it is "too late" to begin? Does a person have to be young to achieve success? There have been hundreds of stories of individuals who joined the ranks of athletes well after what could be considered "too old." Dr. Andrew Weil, [7] in his book, *Healthy Aging: A Lifelong Guide to Your*

47

Well-Being, mentions a couple of Japanese men, a father, Keizo Miura and his son, Yuichiro, who were record-breakers in the grueling physical sport of mountain climbing. The father climbed Mt. Kilimanjaro at seventy-seven in 1981; his son in 2003 climbed Mt. Everest at seventy-two, the oldest man to ever reach the summit.[8] (Yuichiro, when eighty years old, broke his own Everest record in 2013.)

Some cultures live longer than others. The people of Okinawa are a good example, and they do it without formal training. Their daily lives include physical activity such as chopping wood, farming by hand, and carrying water. They walk almost everywhere all their lives. No marathons. Just hard work.

I'll mention one more example of the accomplishments of older athletes: the amazing story of Robert Marchand, born in 1911 in France. My daughter told me she heard about him on NPR while driving to work. Interested, I found a **New York Times** source as well. Marchand was a firefighter in Paris in the 1930s, a prisoner of war (WWII), a lumberjack in Canada, and a wine dealer in France. Though a diminutive man (5 ft., 112 lbs.), he had an affinity for the bicycle and engaged in cycling races when he was in his thirties. In his later life, he stayed in condition on an indoor cycle and decided to try to break age-related records for track cycling. When he was 103 years old, he covered 16.7 miles in one hour on a track. At 105, he did 14 miles in one hour, both **Guinness Book Records**. There is ordinary and then there is extraordinary. No one is too old to get the best from themselves. There is always a better you out there—if that's what you want.

••••••

What does the latest research say?

The Week, a newsmagazine of various topics both domestic and international, was mailed to me free to get me to subscribe. In the March 30 issue, a paragraph on page seventeen caught my eye. The title of the short article was "Exercise Slows Aging." British scientists compared two groups, one of over a hundred cyclists between fifty-five and seventy-nine years old, the other a group of people who did not exercise, including some in their twenties and thirties. The bikers performed better in every tested category: muscle retention, less body fat, balance, and immune function. T cells, which protect against infection, were still being produced by the older group—as much as the twenty-plus-year-olds—whereas the non-exercising group's T-cell production had slowed down significantly. The research strongly suggests that you will stay younger if you stay active. [9]

Strangely enough, another piece of information from a dear friend in San Francisco arrived on this same day. Published in the *New York Times*, it was titled "How to Do the Shortest Workout Possible." It's a one-minute workout. Scientist Martin Gilbala[10] has done the research and discovered that three 20-second bursts of high intensity on an indoor bike with two minutes of slow pedaling may be as effective health-wise as forty-five minutes of normal aerobic workouts. Mr. Gilbala has written a book, *The One-Minute Workout*, which was published in 2017.[11]

••••••

"Believe nothing, no matter where you read it, or who said it, no matter if I said it, unless it agrees with your own reason and own common sense."
— Buddha

Life has no remote. Get up and change it yourself. — Anonymous

Uncertainty is a fact of life — expect it and be prepared to deal with it.
The greatest risk is not taking one.
— AIG (insurance company)

••••••

CHAPTER 4
My Timeline

Back in my father's day, health was something people hoped for but didn't think much about. They either had it or they didn't. I don't remember anyone who exercised for the sake of health. Exercise was a by-product of occupation, if it happened at all. The research just wasn't there.

There was a time when medical doctors who wrote columns saying, in essence, that exercise was completely worthless. There were doctors and scientists who once laughed at Linus Pauling, American chemist and biochemist, when he suggested that large doses of vitamin C had great health benefits.[1] The opinions of the naysayers were, in both cases, dead wrong. Dr. Pauling lived to be ninety-three. Maybe he knew something they didn't. Over time we have discovered that how we live our lives—the lifestyle we choose and the food we eat—has much to do with how we age and how long we live. Or how much life we have in our years, however many.

In my teens and early twenties, I attended Mississippi State University on a track scholarship. Because staying in top shape was something I had to do, health and lifestyle was not something I had to think about. It was like being in prison for four years. All my daytime decisions were made for me. Of course, there is always sundown and a honky-tonk somewhere. But again, my nerdish nature triumphed. I didn't drink a beer until I was thirty. I fear that since then, I might have caught up with the teammates who started much earlier than I did. But that's another story.

In my late twenties. I lived in California, pursuing my dream, writing songs, hoping something good would happen, married, with a small daughter, and gaining weight. Life had moved in, apparently settling in my midsection. My indentured servitude in the college athletic world was only a memory, and I had grown pudgy. I'd put on eighteen pounds, which to some doesn't sound like much, but I didn't like the way I felt or looked. I had acquired what was called back then "love handles." I had to do something.

Against all odds, I started running again. In college, having to do this every day becomes a tedious job. It ceases to be fun. You use profanity a lot, and you say to yourself, I'll never get involved with running or anything resembling it again. But eventually there's a boomerang effect. Perversely, you start to miss it, though you're not really sure why. Many athletes end up going back to the thing they hated most at one point in their lives. Contrary to all my former pronouncements and intentions, I did too.

If nothing else, I knew how to get back into condition. The weather was always great in California, and there were hills to run, paths to bike, and the beach full of bikinis. Hardbodies. A strongly health-minded culture existed there. I lost the weight fairly easily on my own terms without some coach admonishing me to "pick it up." Maybe this was the answer.

And it was, for a while. Like any exercise, it only works as long as it remains interesting. I graduated from running for weight control to adding intervals and entering some races. Now in Nashville in my mid-thirties, I continued to pursue my songwriter dream. I played tennis and church league basketball. As I grew older, the running turned into jogging, a craze that had descended on American culture. So many people back then told me, "I hate jogging. If that's what it takes to lose weight, count me out. I'll diet. Or smoke more. Or start smoking." Jogging also did nothing for quickness on the tennis court. Slow doesn't magically translate to fast.

After several years of being an almost evangelical proponent of jogging, I began to see the naysayers' point. Though I tried hard to stay on the program, my interest had waned as with many repetitive activities. There was also potential structural damage to the joints: hips, knees, and feet (plantar fasciitis—I had it—not fun), and a host of other issues. Eventually, the thought of lacing up my shoes, walking into the winter cold or the summer heat, and pounding the pavement for two to five miles became unbearable. I learned it's hard to keep doing something you dislike and do it voluntarily, much less do it well. I had two choices: let myself slide backwards and hope for the best, which I knew wouldn't work, or find another way to get the same benefits. It was time to find a new interest.

I turned to the bicycle more out of necessity than some epiphany. For someone with knee problems, the bike is a kinder, gentler workout (unless a semi runs you over). And it was more fun, though I could make it as tough and as unfun as I wanted. The downside is that cycling is time-consuming. It takes more time to obtain the same amount of aerobic benefit that running provides. I guesstimated the proportion as three and one-half miles on the bike (15-20 minutes) to one mile of running/jogging (8-10 minutes). But I rode this mechanical horse for a while and ended up doing four Bike Rides Across Tennessee, organized by the Tennessee State Parks department. It sounds a lot more impressive and difficult than it actually was. And it was a hoot. Sixty-five to eighty miles a day for six days with a conglomeration of unrelated people of all shapes sizes, and walks of life: lawyers, doctors, house-wives, songwriters, gear-heads, young Turks, old farts— (I didn't qualify at that time).

I did the first ride across the state, and one of the most memorable, with Johnny MacRae, a dear friend, mentor, and great songwriter. It was 1980 and Carl Lewis and the Olympics were on TV every night. I could buy a whole pizza and a pitcher of beer, share it with my riding buddy, and not gain an ounce. Everyone had a story. One woman, who was not slim and didn't look like an athlete, defiantly told us, "My husband said I couldn't do this." She left every morning early, took her time, and completed the whole ride. Bottom line? Though we all had sore butts, it was a great time.

I can't say cycling is the answer for everyone. It is a dangerous proposition unless it's on a road closed to automobiles. There are still drivers who think:

1) A bike is a toy and should be used on the sidewalk (against the law);

2) Bikes should be ridden facing traffic, not with it (dangerous and wrong); and

3) Bikes don't have the same rights and privileges as an automobile (also untrue). Unless otherwise stated, bikes can do anything a car can do except travel on the freeway. They are like twenty to thirty pound two-wheel cars without a lot of acceleration, and with a top speed of maybe 35 mph. Bikers who are not too smart might hit 50 mph going downhill. And other than the bike helmet, which offers some protection for your head and brain, you have little protection on a bike if you're hit by dogs or cars, if you hit a curb, have a flat, get a tire stuck in a drainage grate, or simply fall because your pant leg gets caught in the chain sprocket! One of the oddest stories I heard was of a snake getting tangled in the front wheel. Biking can be fun—if you can avoid the pitfalls, the dangers.

Eventually, you've ridden every safe local road multiple times, and you have to do more and more elaborate preparations to maintain interest. Some people ride because that's their thing. To me, it was a means to an end, not an end in itself. I never grew to dislike riding, but the time came when I needed something different. And I'd always felt that it took too much time. In the past several years, Nashville has added bike lanes, thus reducing the danger element. But not soon enough for me.

So what to do? Back to running, but with a wrinkle. Instead of the drudgery of jogging three to five miles, I decided on intervals. Shorter distance, higher intensity. Five times two hundred yards (uphill or flat) on a specific interval. Not boring, not as time-consuming. It brought my heart rate to near maximum for my age. Not bad. And it worked for me. My weight didn't fluctuate, and there was an added bonus: I was quicker on the tennis court. Not many of us engage the fast-twitch muscle fibers after a certain age. They atrophy and don't burn calories the way they once did—the use-it-or-lose-it principle. With any high-intensity program, these get a workout.

Somewhere in my forties, I got interested in training with weights. The information was out. You lose muscle mass with time unless you do something about it. Not only do you get weaker, but you don't burn as many calories. Weaker, smaller muscles don't necessarily make you eat less. So you get soft. My goal was to stay as strong as I could for as long as I could, and once I started, I never stopped. It's something we all should do. But I never did two-hour sessions three times a week. I'm not lazy, but I'm also not trying to be a bodybuilder—just to hold my own in the maintaining-strength department.

When I turned fifty, I didn't look back, for as Satchel Paige said: "Somethin' might be gainin' on you." I gravitated toward the game of golf. Tennis eventually became a once-a-week activity during warm weather. My fiftieth birthday was a turning point of sorts. I had never been much on stretching, and consequently, I was physically fit but not very flexible. I couldn't touch my toes. I reached somewhere in the neighborhood of my ankles. I read that Kareem-Abdul Jabbar attributed his being able to play in the NBA until the age of forty-one to practicing yoga. That interested me. I'd always thought it was meditation, granola, chanting, sitar music, and marijuana. Little did I know.

What I did know was that to be a decent golfer, you need flexibility, balance, and strong hands and wrists. Whether your goal is just to slow down the aging train or engage in any kind of athletic endeavor, these are good traits to have. I learned that the ultimate goals of yoga were flexibility, balance, strength, and the alignment of the spine. Yogis believe that a man's age is determined by the flexibility of his spine. After a while, I knew what they were talking about. I first started in a YMCA beginner's class. It was fairly simple, and in addition, everyone there was supportive and non-competitive. I soon learned that it doesn't matter how "bad" you think you are, everyone in the class started in the same place. You are your only competition. The people you're in class with, are an added benefit. Some may end up as your friends, but if not, you will at least have someone to suffer with. It looks easier than it is, and you can make it as challenging as you want.

The time came when I realized I was in a war. We ALL are. The specific age number is an individual thing. For me, it was somewhere in my sixties. I knew I had to fight the relentless tide of aging and its consequences. Not doing so would be surrendering, going downhill prematurely. So if you are on board, congratulations. Welcome to our war. I feel it's the most important thing anyone can do with their time.

As of this moment, I'm still around. I've been able, so far, to duck what looked like my fatal destiny. In 2018, I turned seventy-six. I'm 6'1" and weigh 153 pounds. I take two daily medications: a cheap, generic statin and a baby aspirin. I railed against my doctors about the statin, but I lost that battle. They gave me research that, for the moment, convinced me, albeit grudgingly, that it made more sense to follow their advice than not. I eat well and have never dieted. When I tell people my age, they say, "I never would have guessed." They might be lying or avoiding saying that I look much older, but I'm going to take them at their word. I still play golf and tennis with guys fifteen to twenty years younger and hold my own, if not sometimes win. And every day that I get up and can do some of the physical things I do, I win. That's the reward for doing the work. And stronger and better is within everyone's reach.

••••••

"Eighty percent of success is just showing up." —Woody Allen

••••••

The Aging Train: How _You_ Can Slow It Down

CHAPTER FIVE

Working Out Part I: Obstacles We Face

Obstacle 1, Gravity (Are You Serious?)

In 1981 John McEnroe, in a match against Tom Gullikson, lashed out at the chair umpire with the infamous quote, "You can't be serious. You cannot be serious." I would hazard a guess that the chair umpire, if he had completely ignored British drawing room decorum, might have said, "Mr. McEnroe, as a matter of fact, I'm dead serious." I believe posture should be taken seriously.

Gravity has been working on me all my life. But posture is something I never thought about much until I approached my sixtieth year. I became more aware of how we move. How we carry our bodies speaks silent volumes about us. It's the first message we send when we walk into a room or stop to talk to someone. Most of us who reach a certain age have that hang-dog look—the shoulders are rounded forward, the head, instead of being upright and in a straight line with the spine, is pushed forward, and the neck is turtled out to support it. This posture says, life has whipped me into submission. Life certainly can do that, but we don't have to be a walking billboard advertising it. To many of us, our posture is simply a bad habit reinforced through time. And it's not something we realize. Poor posture may feel normal to us, but it's not optimal. Why? It not only says to others, "I'm old," but the head—which weighs between 8 and 12 lbs.—when not aligned properly puts pressure on the cervical and thoracic spine, potentially resulting in headaches and pain between the shoulder blades. Fixing this is as simple—and difficult—as changing our posture. I suffered this problem until the time a chiropractor friend who knew his business made me aware of my poor posture.

I know some people are skeptical of chiropractors. Up until fairly recently, the American Medical Association (AMA) churned out propaganda saying there was no medical value to chiropractic. Research shows there are health benefits from chiropractic care, and I've experienced them.[1] Practicing chiropractors have to be licensed,[2] which at one time was not the case. There are good and bad chiropractors just as there are good and bad anything. I have been helped enormously by the good ones. A chiropractor's job, in the simplest terms, is to give you a structural tune-up when things get out of whack and to maintain proper alignment once you're back in shape. I've had some naysaying friends tell me that I'll have to keep going for adjustments, that chiropractors never fix what's wrong permanently. I simply tell them that most problems are due to unbalanced activities—golf swings, awkward movements, yard work, and the fact that humans walk erect—which can create vertebral displacement and pain in the back. A chiropractor is not an orthopedic surgeon; there is no "fixing" muscular weakness or congenital anomalies. The field is all about structural maintenance, which is ongoing depending on your physical activities. And in many cases, back surgery, or any surgery, produces more problems than it succeeds in rectifying.

When I began to work on posture, the change was amazing. It very quickly made a difference in how I felt—for one thing, more relaxed and confident. Physically, I felt balanced; I floated instead of trudged. I had more than one friend say, "I know this sounds crazy, but have you grown taller?" It seemed that way. I was seeing the world from a slightly different angle, and for some reason, it looked better. I don't know if this is unique to me, but it's true. Standing tall also silently shouts, Younger! A recent report in the national news said that people who work on flexibility are likely to keep their car keys later in life.[3] Flexibility is necessary for every movement, including those awkward twists that parallel parking a car requires. Move it or lose it— in this case, your freedom to drive a car.

Caveat: While first practicing, correct posture will seem awkward and uncomfortable. It's hard to change something you've been practicing for almost as long as you've been on this earth. Making this change will not be easy, and sliding back to what you used to do will probably happen. But hang in there. Posture is a habit. And good posture—if you don't already have it—is not the habit and feeling you're used to, but it can be changed.

What my chiropractor taught me was the following:

1) Back up to a wall. Put your heels, buttocks, shoulders, and the back of your head against the wall. Your spinal column will be upright, each vertebra in line with the one above and below.

2) When you walk, imagine a string attached to the center of the top of your head, pulling you skyward. You should be relaxed—not tense.

It's that simple. And that difficult. Difficult because it will take quite a while for your new position to feel natural where you don't have to constantly check yourself. But be patient. I believe you'll begin to see the benefits soon, despite the learning curve. Or the unlearning curve, as the case may be. (Or the leaning curve.)

To check yourself, there is another way that doesn't require a wall or mirror. Stand erect and relaxed with your arms down by your side. Reach behind you with both arms and grab your right wrist with your left hand, then pull gently down. It's important to stay relaxed especially your shoulders. You'll feel your shoulders drop back and your neck elongate. You can do this even while walking.

I had a wise in-law who once told me, "We're all handmade." This felt profound in its simplicity. We as human beings have much in common — physically, chemically, and intellectually—but we have great differences as well. Not everyone can take certain medications; some people smoke and never get cancer, some get it from secondhand smoke; some people handle stress well, some don't. As you can imagine, there are countless other examples. The point being, you are the only one who can be your health expert. You are your own experiment, your own research project. I once wrote a little feel-good essay called "The Lesson of The Snowflake" where I compared individual humans to snowflakes (before it became a pejorative term for being a political liberal). We all have similarities, but we're all different when you look at us under the microscope of individuality. As health care becomes more homogenized and "efficient," it's less likely to fit you. One size doesn't fit all, particularly when confronted with the complexity of the human body. Your doctor— even if he or she is old school, knows you, and is a hands-on practitioner—will never completely know the subtleties of the organism that is you. You must learn as much as you can about your unique makeup, weaknesses, and strengths, and dare to experiment with different workouts, different foods, and different ways of living. I've always believed in trying things. If something doesn't work, abandon it. There is an old tennis adage that's applicable to a lot of things: Never change a winning game. Always change a losing game.

······

"The greatest pleasure in life is doing what people say you cannot do."
— Walter Bagehot

"If you are going through hell, keep going."
— Winston Churchill

······

Obstacle 2, Inertia

Inertia is often defined as the tendency of a body to remain at rest or stay in motion unless acted upon by an outside force. That would also apply to humans. Inertia is one of our most persistent foes, and it requires activity and proactivity. Since we are all animals—some of us more than others—we all need some kind of consistent and organized workout program, a battle plan. Will you have passion for the workouts? Maybe not. Do you have to have passion? It would help, but not necessarily—it depends on your nature. The only passion you must have is for your personal goal, whether modest or grand. Few people have a passion for working out hard. Those few, though we may regard them as perverse, are getting something out of it that we might not. I have a good friend, a well-known A-list musician in Nashville, who told me he would sometimes go to Centennial Park after a late recording session and run several miles. When I told him he could get more with a lot less, he said, "There is something Zen-like about running several miles. For me, it's not only about weight loss or being in shape, it's about putting stress in its place. It calms me." Fair enough. We're all different, and we all have different priorities. He knew what was best for him.

The Power of Habit by Charles Duhigg gives a reasonable suggestion.[4] He recommends a conditioning process. If you want to go to the gym on a scheduled day, put your sneakers by the door. After you go, reward yourself. A piece of chocolate something, a night out at the movies. Whatever is motivating for you. Or engage a friend as a workout buddy. It will be harder for you to skip if you have someone counting on you. I'm always amused and annoyed by the New Year's "resolutioneers." They show up in January en masse at the YMCA I attend, making it difficult to find a parking place and a free machine for my workout. But I patiently wait. I know what happens next. They gradually thin out and leave the Y—with a few exceptions—to the diehards. This happens by March or so.

Obstacles 3 and 4, Discipline and Perfectionism

One of the main stumbling blocks to any program, whether it be learning to play the piano, learning a language, or working out, is the discipline required to hang in there and not give yourself excuses not to do the work. Some lucky few have unyielding self-discipline. If you skip, make sure the reason is legitimate and you're not manipulating (BS-ing) yourself. You have to create a habit. If you skipped without a true reason, don't spin it. Admit it. Don't worry about it or feel guilty. We all have those days. Just get back on track tomorrow.

In our culture, we sometimes tell ourselves we need to be great to matter or succeed. It's a classic case of the perfect being the enemy of the good. Perfectionism is a trap. All we can do is compete with ourselves. Everyone has different abilities and limits. There is only one Roger Federer and one Tiger Woods. If I wanted to be a scratch golfer starting at fifty, or a ranked tennis player for my age starting at thirty-five, it would be far beyond my capabilities. My goal was to find my limits and try to achieve something close.

Obstacle 5, The Body We Start With

Whether it is about flexibility, core strength, body mass index (BMI), or any of a host of physical attributes, we all start where we start. Flexibility and core strength are necessary to help in the prevention of back problems, and the back is at the center of all physical activity. Read ahead for an exercise to build flexibility. Core strength is built up over time and yoga is one of the most effective methods for strengthening your core.

As for BMI, it is something we all have to reckon with. Obesity is a complicated subject and it is assigned so much cultural baggage, from the body images promoted in media, to the proliferation of diets and eating disorders, to the judgment and discrimination faced by people struggling with weight-based issues. Obesity has become a global phenomenon, exacerbated in part by processed foods—high-calorie chemical concoctions of fat, sugar, and salt—which are addictive to too many of us. The result of not eating "real" food is that the body doesn't get what it needs. So you may eat more, too much, trying to satisfy the need. There is another insidious player that is not a food: The Internet and the I-Phone, both of which have proven to be highly addictive, leaving little time or inclination towards any physical activity. A perfect storm. To paraphrase Dr. Phil, "How's it working for us?" No matter your challenges, a support team can make all the difference. There are health specialists, coaches, and personal trainers. There are friends, family, a whole tribe of your choosing. We start where we start but we deserve every chance to get where we want to go.

Obstacle 6, Age

I believe age is only as big an obstacle as we make it. I traveled to China in 2008. One of the typical tourist stops is the Great Wall. There were hundreds of people, both international and Chinese tourists, climbing the wall. The Great Wall has steps, but they are not uniform. Some are 2 feet high and some are what we consider normal heights, but they're not that easy for anyone to negotiate. One of the amazing sights I saw was an aged Chinese lady being helped by her daughter to step down the last couple of difficult steps to where I was starting my climb. She had obviously climbed up the Great Wall and, with a little help, descended it. She appeared to be at least eighty if not older. Many people are in wheelchairs at her age. In Beijing one morning, I saw hundreds gathered in Tienanmen Square, doing synchronous Tai Chi. It was quite a sight. It all depends on genetic luck and what you decide to do in life. Age is only as much of an obstacle as you make it.

······

Aging is not for wimps.
—Fred A. (Johnny) MacRae,
A dear friend, no longer with us

······

CHAPTER 6
Overcoming the Obstacles—Strength, Balance, and Flexibility

To age well, you have to address five key fitness areas: strength, balance, flexibility, and aerobic vs. anaerobic workouts. All are important in their own ways. What you do and how you do it depends on your goals and where you are now. If you're completely out of shape, say one notch above (hopefully not below) a couch potato, serious consideration needs to be given to what exercises and how much of each. Where you start is as important as where you want to arrive. Some folks might just want to walk with their dog, and nothing is wrong with that. But understand that this might be the lowest rung on your ladder. It depends on how high you're aiming.

Nautilus equipment was my original strength-building tool. Gyms are full of them. They are machines that isolate and train a muscle, say the bicep, and according to marketing, can build muscles more efficiently, and more safely. That is a matter of opinion. Some of the stations take a lot of the necessity for balance out of the exercise equation. They are, in some cases, useful, but not necessarily the best choice for every muscle or muscle movement. I use the ones where I can trigger multiple muscles with one exercise. Why? In the real world, muscles are used together, rarely solitary, and keeping and practicing balance are important. Best to exercise that way if possible. However, if you want to be great at carrying heavy boxes, or showing off your "big guns," Nautilus curls might be your go-to choice.

After experimenting with the machines, I decided it might make more sense to do a combination of exercises that hit several muscles, making them work together as they may in routine daily situations. Instead of the bicep curl, I decided on pull-ups. (They used to be called "chinning.") You grip a horizontal bar mounted above your head and, with your arms, pull yourself up until your chin is just short or even with the bar. Lower your body and repeat. Why? Think of the muscles you're triggering and strengthening: the biceps, the shoulders, the latissimus dorsi (lats), and the trapezius. Of course, pulling your body weight up with your arms is difficult for most, impossible for some. There is a machine called a Gravitron that provides a counter-weight system allowing users to find the amount of weight they can handle. If your gym doesn't have one, you can always do the Nautilus curl thing until you gain enough strength.

Some Nautilus machines are hard to avoid because they can't be easily replicated unless you use elastic exercise bands. The hamstring machine is one. Dumbbells also have their place. Shoulder raises with light weights are good:

Start with the dumbbells down by your side with your thumbs extended forward onto the bell part. Raise your arms slowly up and at a 45-degree angle diagonal to your body, not straight ahead or out to the side, but between the two positions, and stop 10 degrees short

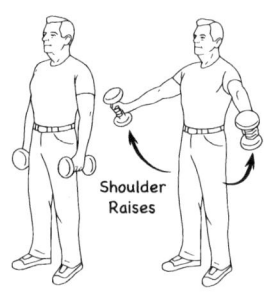

Shoulder Raises

of parallel to the floor. In other words, don't go as far up as the shoulder. As the dumbbells are raised, the thumb should always be pointing up. You can also have a slight bend in the arms if that is more comfortable.

Keep in mind that shoulders are very vulnerable. A physical therapist once told me that with a joint, you can have stability or mobility; you don't get both.

So why my focus on combo exercises? The bonus muscles are triggered and the time involved is shortened. Unless you want to make the Y or the gym your social outlet (which is fine if you do), you can save time. I rarely spend more than twenty minutes in the Y doing my strength routine, twice a week! And I don't feel the shorter time has compromised my strength goals. Like Yoga, it's about strength, flexibility, and balance. And balance applies to life, not just to standing on one foot with your eyes closed. If you're a beginner, I recommend that you engage a trainer who can help you with unfamiliar terms, the equipment, and the proper form. The YMCA and other gym have many competent people who can get you up to speed.

My Workout

1) **I do pull-ups ("chin-ups")** to failure. Starting in 2013, I did seven-eight reps. My first goal was ten reps. I wasn't sure I'd make it. Note: I did ten reps on 4/27/13. I had to do it again to prove it wasn't a fluke, which it might have been. At age seventy-four, 2016, I did eighteen. Now at age seventy-six, on a good day, I do twenty. If you do the work, you will improve.

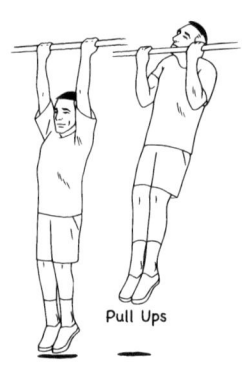

Pull Ups

2) **Triceps Pulldowns.** This requires a Nautilus machine, one that has a bar or rope suspended from above, hooked to a cable. Start with twenty pounds. If it's too easy, increase the weight. Do the opposite if it's too hard. I bend at the waist and basically pull the bar down, triggering triceps,

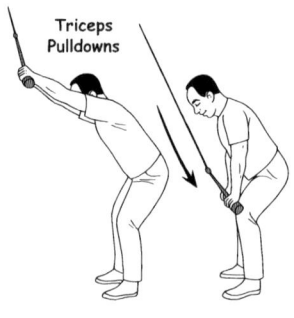

Triceps Pulldowns

lats, shoulders, and stomach muscles, replicating a tennis service motion or throwing a ball. Or you can throw a medicine ball at the floor. (Downside?) It's loud and possibly annoying. Do as many reps as you can. If you go over fifteen, you need to apply more weight. At first, I was only able to do four-five to failure. Now I'm using 77.5 lbs. and now able to do reps in the teens.

3) **One more set of Number 1** (pull-ups).

4) **One more set of Number 2** (triceps pulldowns). I usually alternate between the pullups and the pulldowns.

5) **Crunches on an exercise ball.** (A crunch is an abdominal exercise. While lying on the floor or on an exercise ball, lift your shoulders toward your pelvis using your stomach muscles—hence the word "crunch.") Make sure you hit all the abdominals by rolling the ball toward your buttocks, which hits the lower abs. Make sure you are close to a fixed pole or a wall for balance. I do one hundred to 125 most of the time. One set.

Crunches on Exercise Ball

6) **Two sets of shoulder raises.** This exercise was mentioned earlier. Start with dumbbells in each hand down by your side. Raise the weights with your shoulders, not swinging, but by lifting with straight arms upward or with a slight bend. I stop

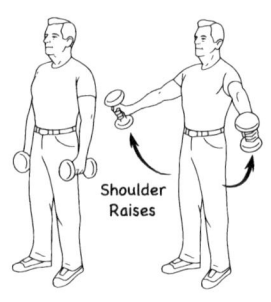

Shoulder Raises

6 inches short of horizontal. Rotate your wrists with thumbs up and splay the arms out at a 45-degree angle. Use a light weight and do fifteen to twenty reps. You should be feeling tired by then. I never rest to get to the second set. For variety and balance, I do half the reps on one foot and then switch. I always do some other exercises to target different muscles in between sets. I like active rest. It saves time and keeps the metabolism up.

7) **Shoulder shrugs.** Dumbbells in hand, raise your shoulders toward your ears. Twenty reps. One set. Follow this with what is called the Farmer's Walk: With the same dumbbells, hands down at your side, walk 20 steps away from the rack and then turn and go back. I use two 70-lb. dumbbells. Caution: This is a lot of weight, but I've been doing this for years and know my limits. I suggest you start with two 25-lb. dumbbells or lower. Find your level, and let the weight grow naturally.

8) **Torso rotation.** This is a Nautilus machine that targets the abs and core. It's a great core builder. Since I do other exercises, I only do one set of this on each side. It helps with one of our greatest problems,

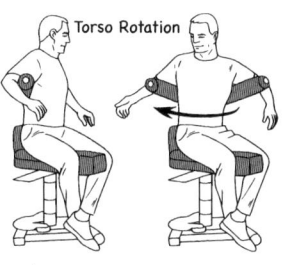

Torso Rotation

muscle imbalance. Since few of us are ambidextrous, we overbuild one side of our body, which can lead to back and hip problems.

9) **Hamstring curls.** Another Nautilus machine. Facedown on the padded bench. You hook your ankles under a pad and pull your heels toward your bottom, using your hamstrings, the muscles behind your thighs. Use light weights until you determine where you are. I do only one set, and I do it because I have to sprint in tennis. Weak or unconditioned hamstrings can be injured. It's painful and slow to heal. It is one of the most common injuries when a football player comes back from the summer hiatus and starts to sprint. Remember the cardinal rule of any exercise: Avoid injury.

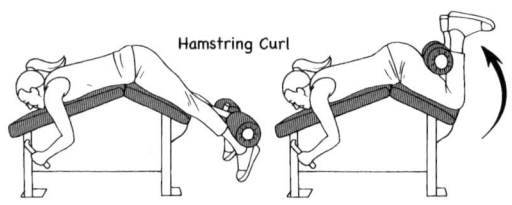

Hamstring Curl

10) **Adduction/Abduction**—Adduction is building the muscles on the inside of our thighs that allow us to pull our legs together against resistance. The easiest to use is a Nautilus machine if you have access. It targets muscles that are hard to get to unless you use elastic exercise bands.

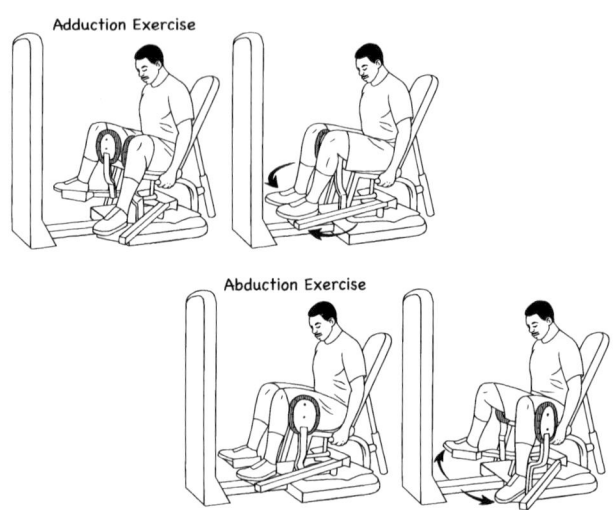

Adduction Exercise

Abduction Exercise

Abduction is the opposite. These are muscles on the outside, the hip, and thigh, and they allow you to push your legs outward against resistance. Both sets of muscles are important for tennis players or anyone who uses their legs in a sport. They're not as important for walkers.

11) **Lunges.** (If you have knee issues, which many of a certain age do, consult your doctor or physical therapist before attempting this exercise.) A lunge is basically, "taking a knee." Start with your feet together. Take a long step

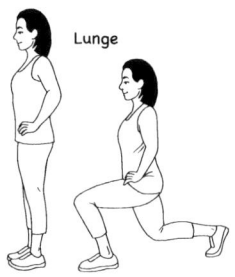
Lunge

forward with the right leg and slowly lower your body, keeping your posture erect and balanced until the forward leg is parallel to the floor. Slowly raise your body and place the back foot on the left, even with the forward. Then step forward with the left foot and repeat. Lunges are not for everyone. If you can do them, they are one of the great combination exercises. They target quads and gluteal muscles, they challenge balance, and if you want to hold a dumbbell in a curl position or do curls simultaneously, they work even more muscles. A good substitute exercise is half squats with or without dumbbells. As before, never go below thigh being parallel to the floor. Easier on the knees.

I'm not a huge fan of leg presses or squats, though they do have some use, particularly for younger athletes. I'm also not a fan of bench presses. I'd recommend pushups instead. They accomplish pretty much the same thing and don't put the same awkward stresses on the shoulders.

I always go from one exercise to another without any pauses. This keeps the heart rate up and again cuts down on time.

Sidestory

Charlie Monk, aka The Mayor of Music Row—a well-known personality in the Nashville music scene—is someone I've known for forty years. He's an all-around good guy and, like all guys, we rib each other. I've never seen him speechless. Ever. My songwriter brain came up with some nicknames: The Yoda of Yakkery? The Grand Poobah of Palaver? The Undisputed Lord of Loquacity? The Consigliore of Confabulation? (I think I just went a bridge too far.) I saw him the other day at the YMCA, talking, as usual, with a friend. He's got a million of them. He was sitting on the seat of a Nautilus station for chest presses. Just sitting. Gabbing away, doing nothing on the machine. I walked over to him, interrupted his conversation, and asked, "What's this exercise called? Interval bullshitting?" (The nice thing about writing this is that Charlie won't have the opportunity to give me a well-aimed verbal riposte—or insult. Score: Bob 1—Monk 0. He will get even, however. He usually does)

Finding Your Balance

With age, balance, like most things, deteriorates. And it is amazing how many ways balance affects us. When playing tennis, you have to change direction often. A while back a doctor asked me if I had fallen yet. I almost said, "No, but should I try to?" It's no joke, however, that the number one cause of accidental death among the elderly is falling.[1] A simple exercise might help your balance:

Try to stand on one foot for one minute, close to a chair or wall to catch yourself if you start to fall. Change to the other foot and do the same thing.

This is not easy. If you think you're terrible at it, you'll have company, believe me. But you'll get better, and this simple exercise might prevent a fall one day. It matters in much the same way as posture does. Very simple, yet important. You can do this exercise while watching TV or waiting for your coffee or tea to brew.

If you want to simplify things and not compromise what you're after, find and join a good Yoga class. A beginner's class is fine if you've not done Yoga in the past or if you haven't done it for a long time. It's an as-difficult-as-you-want-to-make-it, all-encompassing workout that provides most of what you need, including potential social relationships. I highly recommend it. It works on strength, balance, and flexibility. It aids in good posture. Though I think it's a great idea in many ways, I don't do it as often as I should. I do too many other physical activities and, because yoga by itself is a strenuous workout, I wouldn't have enough energy to do that and my personal regimen. I do, however, stretch to maintain flexibility—one characteristic of appearing and feeling younger.

Most teachers suggest going to yoga three times a week, minimum. Depending on age and conditioning, that's probably a good rule of thumb. As with anything, don't be discouraged at what you can't do—be grateful for what you can do. It's a slow process. Think of how many years it took your body to get weak and inflexible. You can't reverse that overnight. People who attend Yoga classes are usually very supportive and non-competitive. And remember that everyone in your class had to start where you did.

Ultimately, balance applies to life, not just to stand on one foot with your eyes closed. If you're a beginner, I recommend that you engage a trainer who can help you with unfamiliar terms, the equipment, and the proper form. The YMCA and other gym have many competent people who can get you up to speed.

••••••

"Life is like riding a bicycle. To keep your balance, you must keep moving." Albert Einstein

••••••

Flexibility and Core

Because I have difficulty scheduling around yoga classes, I now do other stretching to keep my spine flexible, one which I note below. I usually do this when I'm waiting for my coffee to brew. It sounds silly, but I haven't had any serious back issues since I started this:

The broomstick twist: Feet eighteen inches apart. Take a broomstick or a 5-foot or 6-foot wooden dowel, curtain rod, or whatever similar item you have around the house and place it centered on the back of your neck,

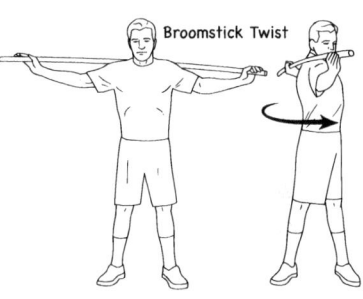

Broomstick Twist

over your shoulders, and drape your arms over it. It's best to have them stretched out, but if the pole is too short, drape them over the pole, bending them at the elbow. Look straight ahead and start twisting your torso and shoulders, rotating the hips gently back and forth. Do thirty to forty reps, fifteen or twenty on each side. When your back begins to loosen toward the latter part of the exercise, maybe the last five or six reps, twist a little farther, trying to increase your flexibility. Never force anything. It's important to keep your head straight, which rotates and increases the flexibility of your neck at the same time. This exercise works the hips, the torso, and the neck. You should see your arm pointing straight in front of you when you rotate ninety degrees from where you started. If not, that's your first goal.

A variation on this exercise came from a fellow golfer whose physical therapist had suggested the one I just described.

Bent Over Stick Twist: Bend over 90 degrees from the waist so that the torso is parallel to the floor, keep a flat back and from that position rotate the shoulders the same way as the original exercise.

The pole will end up pointing more toward the ceiling. It's tough, but it works the hips more.

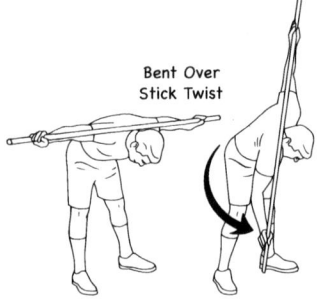

Bent Over
Stick Twist

Give it time. If you can get past that ninety-degree angle and over toward the opposite shoulder, give yourself a smiley face sticker. That means you have better flexibility. (For other exercises like this one, visit The MacKenzie Method online.) [2]

There is no workout that fits everyone. The workout I've described here is what I do for my particular needs. Feel free to substitute or include your favorite exercises. As you age, every day is different. Some days you'll kill the workout, and it will seem easy. Some days it kills you, and everything is an effort. Just do what you can, and in the immortal words of Bob Dylan, "Don't think twice, It's all right." Some things will work that you didn't expect to, and the reverse is also true. Life is not a scripted event. Approach it as though it's an adventure.

The Fitness-Tracking Phenomenon

The basic idea of digital activity tracking is a good one. Track the number of steps you take daily. It gives the user a target to shoot for—ten thousand. My wife started with the basic gadget and enjoyed the feedback. My only problem with it then was its price. For those who already own a relatively sophisticated cell phone, there are numerous apps online that work just fine, some of which can be downloaded free or for a few bucks. Fitbit's greatest advantage, in my opinion, is its small size. Some models are worn on the wrist. Others can be put in your pocket or clipped to your clothes. Originally, I thought the only way it would be of use would be to see how many steps I was taking during a tennis match. Other than that, I wasn't really sold on the gadget. That was my first opinion on the subject. But my wife recently got a newer model, and in all fairness, it's an interesting wrinkle. She likes it even more than the original. I have to admit, it's pretty cool. For those who are interested in stats and gadgets, it's a step up. It not only tracks how many steps you took and the stairs you climbed each day, but it also records your resting heart rate, your maximum heart rate, and the quality and time of your sleep. It then downloads all this data to your computer. Capturing a wide range of information has changed my mind, and I may end up getting a version for myself.

This next suggestion may be strange or controversial, but it is related to maintaining strength and balance and it is not about being an athlete. I've known a lot of couples who chose to sell their house because it had stairs and they, with age, aching knees, and stiff joints, felt a one-story house would work better for them. My wife, Barbara, and I still have a three-story house. The main floor, a working basement downstairs, and a room upstairs where we watch television. It is our choice to walk up and down stairs every day for as long as we can do it. We're now in our mid-seventies, and sometimes it's not easy, but it preserves muscle in the glutes and quads. Fortunately, we have handrails on all three stairways, which I recommend. You would be amazed at how many floors you can climb and how many steps you can take just around the house. It's like a low-impact workout on its own. Without realizing it, we've joined a whole new movement called "aging in place." I'm aware that some folks have disabilities or other issues where having stairs makes no sense. But I've always felt that as we age, we have to challenge ourselves wherever we can, within reason. This is not for everybody. It's your choice, as is everything on these pages.

CHAPTER 7
The Secrets to Efficient Exercise - Intensity and Intervals

The Secret of Intensity

If your goal is to lose a substantial amount of weight, walking it off might take far too long to make that a reasonable choice. If you're a seventy-year-old man who wants to hit a golf ball 230 yards or be able to run down a wide forehand and topspin it down the line, walking won't achieve these things. You'll need more effort, but, amazingly, NOT MORE TIME. That's the shocking part. To people who say they don't have time, I can tell you that four intense minutes is all it takes for the metabolic rate to remain raised for at least thirty minutes after the workout. And maybe longer, though there is disagreement about the actual length of the calorie burn. I know that sounds too good to be true, but it hasn't been for me.

So, one secret to turning back the body's clock is working out with intensity. I had always found a way to do my workouts outdoors. But looking for a different way to train other than biking and jogging, I started going to the gym more often. I tried alternating Nautilus for muscle and strength retention with indoor biking for aerobic conditioning. I called it my intense workout. Two Nautilus stations, one set on each, and then I would go immediately to an indoor bike and pedal for three minutes, one minute hard, one minute rest or slow pedaling, and one minute hard again. Then back to the Nautilus stations for the final of two sets. Then I'd do the bike and move on to another pair of stations. I would never rest long enough to have my heart rate return to normal. That way, it was almost constant motion. I did this sequence twice a week. It didn't take that long, but it was not easy. The one thing I learned from it is that I enjoyed the short intense workout a lot more than a long slow one. I was to learn later that the benefits are multiplied when we work out this way. The metabolism is kicked up into a higher gear and continues to burn fat for several hours. Much more bang for the buck, considering time spent and the results that followed. It's what you do and how hard you do it, not how much time you spend.

The Secret of Intervals

So, what is an "interval"? In simple terms, an interval is alternating a period of high-intensity exercise followed by a period of low intensity or rest. But it's on the clock. Let's say you are going to use an elliptical trainer. After a warmup, you start running or walking as fast as you can for thirty seconds, then back off for a minute. You repeat the process until you reach your goal, whether it be a certain heart rate or a predetermined number of repetitions, or feel like you've had enough.

Make your first interval training simple. If you haven't done much physically in years, understand that it will be difficult at first. There's no quick fix. It's a process. Too many people don't follow through because they want immediate results. It took time to get out of condition, and if that's where you are, it will take time to get back into condition. But not as long as it took you to get out. Realize that if you do something at a physical level beyond your normal level, you will get sore. I'll repeat: you will get sore. Unused muscles are giving you a message, and the message hurts. But relatively soon, if you continue to do the work, the soreness will subside and it will get better. If you're totally out of condition, I'd suggest starting with walking. If you're already walking, try doing intervals uphill. Find a challenging hill close by if possible. Walk fast to a predetermined point that has some difficulty, and then turn around and walk downhill. Assess how you feel.

You can make this an interval workout by giving yourself a time within which to complete each uphill, downhill cycle. The faster you complete the cycle, the more 'recovery' time you can enjoy before the interval starts again. As long as you feel like you can do one more, do it. When it's starting to get really difficult, stop. It takes a few times to know how much is enough or too much for you. Once you start to feel too comfortable, it's time for the next level. Do more repetitions or work out longer or faster, or do a little of each, your choice. Make sure you keep tabs on your exercise heart rate, and adjust the beats per minute (bpm) up or down to fit your needs.

Tabata – High Intensity meets Interval Training

A Japanese researcher, Izumi Tabata, compared the results of anaerobic high-intensity workouts with more traditional aerobic style jogging or walking programs.[1] The conclusions were amazing to me. The anaerobic workouts, in almost all categories, outdid the aerobic workout participants. Fat burning, peak oxygen uptake (VO2), etc. My stumbling onto a more intense workout was an accident. A Tabata workout is only four minutes long, not counting a short warm-up. It requires one to do twenty seconds of maximum effort followed by ten seconds of rest eight consecutive times. Each round is twenty seconds hard plus ten seconds easy which equals thirty seconds eight times which adds up to four minutes total. The ultimate goal is to hit a maximum heart rate, (two hundred twenty, minus your age—I'm seventy-six, my maximum rate is one hundred forty-four). Your baseline physical condition will determine how much of the workout you can do. Understand that being able to do this workout is the top of the mountain, and not recommended for everybody. There are other fewer ways to reach your goals.

Tabata is like the programs referred to in count-less articles and books as HIIT, which is an acronym for "High-intensity interval training." Tabata, however, is "Super High-Intensity Interval Training. "SHIIT" is my acronym for it. It's what I say under my breath (or more accurately under my gasp) when I've just finished the sixth go around. Only two more to go.

If you already have a degree of fitness, try one twenty-second burst of something—indoor bike, a sprint outdoors, elliptical trainer—and stop. Follow the program in the previous paragraph. Alternately, you can start out walking fast on an elliptical trainer, stop for ten seconds, and do it again until you can do eight consecutive reps. You can either do it more intensely and quit when you feel you can't go on, or you can do each interval slowly, gradually increasing the effort until you reach your maximum effort. What you're after is building up to where you can do each twenty seconds at your maximum. The great thing about this kind of workout is that although you're working hard, you don't work long. You don't burn tons of energy in the pursuit of mediocre results. For further information, Google Tabata Protocol.

A Case for Caution

You should consult with your doctor as to whether you are healthy enough to, at some point, work out this rigorously. And if you want to try it, this is important:

you have to begin slowly. Aim for an exercise heart rate of say, one hundred bpm at first. For you, this may be too much or too little. Unless you're a gadget person, there's no need to buy a heart rate monitor. (Some aerobic machines have a built-in heart rate monitor, but they're often inaccurate.) A watch or clock with a second hand will do. Just count the number of your heartbeats for six seconds, and then add a zero to that number. In other words, if you count ten beats in six seconds, the bpm. is one hundred. That's approximately how many times your heart would beat if you counted for the entire minute.

There are many ways to achieve a high heart rate that will continue to burn calories. Exhaustion is not the goal. It's to be avoided, if possible. There will be times you will feel that way. As you improve your condition, recovery will be quicker. There is another benefit to the short, intense workout. Because it's short, it doesn't seem to wear on your joints the way longer, more repetitive workouts do—jogging on concrete for example.

You might be wondering how much time it takes to do my various routines. My strength-building workout is done twice a week and takes about twenty minutes. I go to the YMCA on Wednesday, Saturday, or Sunday, depending on what else is going on. One Tabata workout, including warmup and cooldown, takes about six minutes. I sometimes do more than one. Maybe one and a half or two on days when I'm feeling frisky. My heart rate usually ends up around 145 bpm. I usually try to do two to three Tabatas a week, coupling it with the strength workout or not.

My Tabata choices are jumping rope (for tennis footwork), Kettle Bell swings (for glute and core strength—the toughest one I do), and elliptical trainer sprints (again for tennis and general conditioner). I also occasionally do the stationary bike. If you're a masochist, try the rower. It's one of the toughest. I play tennis and/or golf a couple of times a week when possible. I don't count that as a workout. I do strength training twice a week. I never double up on intense or difficult workouts because there's no benefit. I'm not trying to be a world-class athlete. Just a world-class senior.

You must understand, however, that getting in shape to do something like this will take months of working up to it, especially if you're starting from scratch. But I guarantee this: If you follow through and can end up doing it at whatever level you are capable of, you'll never regret it. You'll feel better, be healthier, and not only will you feel younger and act it, but your body will also be younger. Even though the work gradually gets harder as you go, it feels easier because you'll become accustomed to what the work requires. You'll know what it feels like and you'll know you can handle it. You'll have gotten past the mental roadblock, which is the thing that typically derails most of us who want to move beyond our comfort zone.

The 3rd and Best Secret is the Pay-off

Sure, the long-term outcomes are their own payoff – better health, more vibrant and active living. But there is a short-term payoff too, and it surprises most folks. Exercise gives you energy. It kick-starts your metabolism. When I'm feeling sluggish, the urge is overwhelming to lie on the couch and vegetate. Nothing wrong with that—sometimes. But more often than not, I don't regain any energy by resting. If, against all my inclinations, I force myself to do a couple of minutes of jumping rope or squat jumps, I feel better. Never worse. The difficulty is always in overcoming inertia and a reluctant mind. Which may be redundant.

If whatever regimen you choose is enjoyable and helps you keep your weight in a healthy range, keeps you strong, raises your heart rate, and gives you energy, that's great. Consistency is the key. Playing tennis, biking, hiking, or anything that you'll enjoy—that's the ultimate goal. There is no one road. You just have to have to look for and find your best road. It all boils down to what you want. If you want to lose fat, you have to kick your metabolism in the rear so that it continues to burn even at rest. That means a high-intensity workout. Walking is a great low-impact workout, but it lacks the necessary intensity for fat burning. Understand that high intensity means something different for everyone. What is relatively easy for me may not be possible for you. What is easy for someone else might be impossible for me. All you have to do is find your level and build on it.

CHAPTER 8
Food for Thought - What We Eat and Why It Matters

Right now, at a laboratory somewhere, chemists are experimenting with different combinations of fat, sugar, and salt —major components of processed foods. There is no consideration given to the result of consuming these products, only to how they taste. They are concocted to taste great. We all know that. But they are nothing but man-made chemical compositions. They give nothing but a moment's pleasure. Because having digested these empty calories, the body then asks for more food, still looking for something it needs. The percentage of overweight and obese people in the U.S. is higher than in most developed nations. We lead the world in the total number of obese people.[1] Shoppers at the cheaper corporate food stores are most at risk and many live in "food deserts" where fresh fruits and vegetables are hard to come by. The resulting health crises are a disaster for them, their families and quite possibly for our whole society. It could well be the reason our nation may never be able to pay for health care for all.

The people who need to stretch their dollars trying to find the cheapest version of food they can. No one can blame them. They are victims of circumstance and a lack of knowledge. It is easy to forget that the availability of healthy food correlates directly to the extent of privilege in a given neighbor-hood. I was lucky not to be caught in the revolving door of poverty. But unfortunately for those who are, it's a pay-me-now or pay-me-later scenario. The money someone saves on processed junk today is nowhere near the money they or others will spend on the negative health consequences that occur as they age. Statistically, they will age quicker, look older, and get sick and/or die sooner. We tend to be a culture that does not pay attention to tomorrow. We focus on the moment. Not a good choice for our health, because tomorrow will come. And quicker than we think. Every country's population in the world that has experienced the introduction and growth of American fast food outlets begins to gain weight. So, it's not just us. It's not a lack of willpower. It's our bodies silently screaming for what they need.

Some Backstory

There's a history of how our food supply has been compromised. In brief: Richard Nixon appointed a man by the name of Earl Butz to be the agriculture chief in 1971. Johnny Carson used to have a field day with that name, as you can imagine. Butz was a bald, gnomish-looking shill of Big Ag. His opinion was that the U.S. should corporatize the entire food system, basically telling individual farmers to fall in line or go under financially.2 So much for freedom and individualism. This led to a flood of corn-based products. I'll name just two: ethanol, and the most pervasive and one of the most harmful food additives in history—high fructose corn syrup (HFCS). Since then, year after year, the number of family farms continues to dwindle, at the time of this writing down to 2.1 million from an original high of over 6 million.3 It might be an even lower number by the time you hold this book in your hands. With one year of drought, or too much rain, or any other weather-related catastrophes, that number will diminish because individual farmers can't withstand more than a season or two of failed crops. Corporations do. They have deep pockets and subsidies and the political power to ensure the status quo.

Engineered corn is like an evil Santa Claus—it's everywhere. To give the reader some perspective, at one time there were thirty different varieties of corn—many indigenous to Mexico. Through chemical manipulation, and subsidies that allowed U.S. corn to be sold cheaper than it can be grown, other countries couldn't compete with ours. That made the playing field smaller and more concentrated, designed to create a quasi-monopoly. There are now only six varieties of corn, and big chemical companies are working hard (i.e., paying politicians off) to see that they control it all.[4] Monsanto's seeds are not only chemically "engineered" to grow in the presence of Roundup (active ingredient: isopropylamine salt of glyphosate), which is a carcinogen, but they are also engineered not to reproduce so that seeds will have to be purchased every year instead of reproducing themselves as in nature.

Based on much research, ethanol is as expensive to produce, in terms of energy, like gasoline, and it doesn't work as a viable additive to gasoline to reduce our dependence on foreign oil.[5] I've yet to hear someone say, "I'm using this new ethanol-laced fuel and my mileage has really improved . . . isn't science great?" That's because no one can say it. Ethanol also has an insidious habit of fouling and ruining small engines. So much for that corn experiment. But the government keeps sending out the subsidies for Big Ag corn.

Around 1980 our food supply was dealt what could be considered a near-fatal blow by allowing corn to be grown with little governmental regulation—farmers were once required to store excess corn in silos. Chemists were told to find uses for this tidal wave. This gave rise to processed foods full of cheap corn-based chemicals such as high fructose corn syrup. It turned our food supply into little more than junk.[6] It's engineered to taste good, and admittedly, it does. But the body is pretty smart. It knows when it's not getting nutrients, so it asks for more, hoping we'll accidentally shovel something down that will satisfy its needs. But unless you eat real foods with real nutritional value, you will gain weight or become malnourished. You can't go against nature and maintain good health. People who are overweight aren't necessarily gluttons with no will power. Weight gain can be a reaction to a body in need of nutrition. This results from a combination of unawareness, clever marketing, and the wrongheaded idea that if it tastes good, it must be good. Processed food products are not designed to satisfy your hunger. They are designed to make you want to eat more.[7] Our food companies have perfected the perfect product: foodless food!

I used to believe that most companies took into consideration their customers' welfare and would never knowingly do anything detrimental. I now feel, in some cases, that's wishful thinking. Take, for example, the food recalls that seem to be getting more and more prevalent. In many of those cases, someone knew the truth but kept quiet, hoping for the best—that it would either remain undiscovered or would quietly go away. Whistleblowers routinely get vilified and/or fired for doing what they believe is right. "No good deed goes unpunished," though a cliché, is often frighteningly accurate. That's why we individuals have to do our own policing. I'm not happy with that, but there's not much choice.

I know I might sound like some pretentious food-ie (I'm originally from Mississippi, how could I be?), but ask any great chef if you can make great dishes without great natural ingredients. You would hear a unanimous no. The second, more important, reason is that fresh, properly grown organic produce has more nutritional value than most conventional store produce. (Big Ag will tell you otherwise.) Because it's grown in rich, nutrient-filled soil and not in a dead zone of the three chemicals we call fertilizer (nitrogen, potassium, and phosphorus), it contains more trace elements and more natural food quality. There are Big Ag types who will say "This is a charlatan speaking" or "Is this guy a scientist?" or "What could a songwriter know?" Or they'll say, "We have our own people who can, with our own research, completely refute everything he is claiming." Yadda yadda. Are these the same experts that used to work for the tobacco companies? Maybe their sons? Just kidding, but I do think a lot of us have heard this song or some version of it before. Granted, this is all just my scientific opinion but we have to keep in mind that it is in Big Ag's best interest to refute anything that might curtail sales.

How does all this affect us? No one is sure yet, and that's the problem—NO ONE IS SURE. I don't want to eat something conjured up in some corporate chemist's test tube. And I don't care how safe the company says these abominations of nature are. I won't eat them. GMO's—genetically modified organisms—are being banned in Europe and Japan.[8] In the U.S., the chemical companies lobbied hard to not be required to label processed food as a GMO. That tells me all I need to know. They ended up winning, by the way. No surprise there. Bottom line? Avoid processed foods whenever possible. And definitely don't use processed foods that aren't labeled "NO GMOs." Why encourage these guys by contributing to their bottom line?

FYI—There was a time when farmers could take the seeds out of their harvest, dry them, and plant them the next year. That day is over, for the most part. There is a seed storage facility—the Global Seed Vault— in Svalbard, Norway, which is often referred to as the "doomsday vault."[9] It was built in 2008. It's a backup system of every seed in the world, perhaps to guard against mass starvation and the potential extinction of humans after a world-wide crisis—nuclear war, for example, or cat-astrophic weather-related disasters. Many varieties of the foods we once consumed have disappeared. The vault is a grim reminder of the fragile nature of both the world's unstable political landscape and the only planet we're sure we can live on.

A Case for Organic

Organic? I know. I hear you. Organic vegetables and meats cost more. A lot more, in some cases. And it's difficult for most of us to believe that some-thing that costs a lot more but looks the same as something that costs less can possibly be worth the difference. It's simple economics—it's harder to grow organic produce or produce organic animals. Not only is there a smaller market, but it takes more time and costs more money to grow organic. The growers, for the most part, are individual farms, not corporations. I know what some of you say. An apple is an apple is an apple. That makes sense on the surface, and I'd like to agree with you, but I can't. I picked "apple" for a specific reason. Pesticides. They are sprayed to keep insects off, and eating inorganic apples means consuming toxic residue. And though I mention the apple first because it's one of the worst, there is a laundry list of foods good at accumulating pesticides and other undesirable chemicals.

"The Dirty Dozen," [10] according to more than one source, consists of these fruits and vegetables:

Apples

Spinach

Nectarines

Grapes

Peaches

Cherries

Pears

Tomatoes

Celery

Potatoes

Sweet bell peppers

(I have also heard that other sources mention coffee, milk, cheese, butter, and eggs.)

You must consider any fruit or vegetable with thin porous skin. In the same way, your human skin will absorb whatever you apply to it, the apple skin does much the same thing. When we consume even minute amounts of pesticides, they accumulate in the body. The body doesn't know what to do with them. Evidence indicates that cancer is a man-made disease. Only one tissue sample from an Egyptian mummy out of the hundreds examined was found to contain cancer cells.[11] It makes me wonder how many of our health problems are directly linked to the pollution of our world.

In addition to health considerations, another reason to buy organic is how it tastes. People who haven't been told about what they are consuming in our home ask where we got the food on the table. My wife is a great cook, but the ingredients make all the difference. Instead of being fertilized and treated with pesticide to make the plant grow quickly, an organic product is allowed to grow at the pace nature intended, developing its full flavor potential.

While there are many places to buy what's labeled organic produce, it always depends on the sources—are they really organic or organic in name only? If you want to see a good documentary, I earlier recommended Food, Inc. It was nominated for an Oscar in 2010. For years my wife and I have contracted with a CSA (Community-Supported Agriculture and you can find information about your local CSAs online). This is an individual group of farmers who grow organic produce and sell meats raised the old-fashioned way—no antibiotics—like grass-fed beef. Currently, our CSA is an Amish farm, and you can't get more old-fashioned than that. They use no pesticides, no fertilizer. The produce is grown in soil that still has micronutrients. The first strawberries of the season are sweet and delicious. Organic produce tastes better to me and is less expensive than you'd think, and everything is grown with love and respect. We're lucky. But farmers' markets are good sources too. Just investing in organic is a green and sustainable choice. Big Ag would like to run the whole food show, but so far it hasn't been able to. Support your local farmers. Please support your local farmers.

Eating Today for a Better Tomorrow

There is an important food component in the battle against aging. This is not about a diet where you deprive yourself of calories. It's about what choices you make for the calories your body needs. If you want to lose weight, that requires certain activities and lifestyle changes. The changes won't be as difficult if you embrace the idea of change. Most of us have to be dragged kicking and screaming into a new paradigm, a new set of habits. But those who put in the work will be amazed at how adaptable our taste buds are. If you give fresh organic produce and grass-fed meats a fair chance, you will start seeing—and tasting—the benefits of a natural, unprocessed diet.

The only way you'll know something works is if you make a change and give it a chance. Then watch for feedback. Do you feel better? Is your food satisfying? What do you do to make it better suited to your unique chemistry? It's an odd thing, human chemistry. It matters. Changes are often hard at first. But once you taste natural food and see the benefits, you'll never turn back. You'll look better, feel better, and be able to ward off some of the ravages of aging. Food is the best medicine. You are what you eat. We've all heard those phrases, and I'll be the first to admit that I didn't think about them much until I began to do some research on the subject. These are not just cute phrases; there is something to them. Some people believe them, others don't, and others like Scarlett in **Gone With The Wind**, will "think about it tomorrow." But today is always the best day to start anything.

Timing Matters

Sometime in February 2018, **NBC Nightly News** had an intriguing report on a woman who, by restructuring her eating schedule, lost a lot of weight.[12] In the report, she initially weighed 250 pounds. The first thing she did was change her diet to fresh, real food, not skipping any food groups, but skipping the fast or junk varieties. She lost forty pounds. But the next ten pounds were just not coming off on what most would consider a normal eating schedule. According to the NBC report, the University of Alabama in Birmingham had researched time-restricted eating—limiting your food intake to just eight hours. In other words, eating your three meals between 8 a.m. and 4 p.m. It works, according to researchers, because the food is digested and metabolized (three to five hours) by bedtime, and the body, not having to deal with a late meal, burns fat while you sleep. The lady got her inspiration from the research, but she cut the hours during which she ate down to six, from eight a.m. to two p.m. Eventually she started working out at the gym, maintaining her diet, and avoiding sweet drinks—sodas and such. Instead, she drank black coffee or water. I don't know what she weighed at the end of her journey, but she looked as though she'd lost at least one hundred pounds.

In hindsight, I realize the serendipity of my own meal schedule. My wife has never liked late dinners, preferring to eat before six p.m., which to some may smack of the "early-bird special" of senior citizens. Our choice was made not with regard to the potential for gaining weight when you go to bed "full" —that hadn't yet been discovered—but because it wasn't conducive to good sleep. So it seems it's not only what you eat, but when. It gives those who struggle with weight another option in what has turned out to be a crisis, not only here in America, but globally.

A Few Food Lessons I've Learned

I have a morning ritual. The first thing I do is take about 10 ounces of warm water in a glass and add a tablespoon and a half of lemon or lime juice. I drink it through a straw. (It can eat away your tooth enamel if you drink it every day directly from the glass. It's an acid. But so are all citrus fruits and sodas.) My wife keeps a jar of freshly squeezed lemon or lime juice in the fridge, but not necessarily for the Vitamin C. We drink it because it's alkaline in the body. And that seems odd, because lemon juice, as you know, is an acid, but it becomes alkaline when metabolized. The drink has several positive effects. It strengthens the immune system, starts your day with a liquid that aids digestion, balances pH, fights hunger cravings, is a natural diuretic, and even may help clear your skin.[13] A win-win. But drink it through a straw, and afterward swirl fresh water around in your mouth to clean any juice that might cling to your teeth.

There is a strong opinion in Healthland that an alkaline body resists the growth of cancers, and conversely, an acidic body abets it. True? I can't say. But there is no reported harm in drinking lemon juice daily. Many believe this. There have been claims of inhibiting, if not killing, cancer by eating foods that transform the body into an alkaline state. Most of what Americans eat and enjoy, however, like meat and sugar, create an acidic condition. Many vegetables aid in alkalinity. Remember, you don't have to be perfect. Just keep taking small steps in the right direction.

I love my coffee. It's a part of my morning ritual. I use a mild bean from Costa Rica that I've been able to drink every day and not get tired of. Black. No cream, sugar, or additives. Research on coffee (over fifty studies!) tried to prove it was harmful for you. But thus far, current research has shown coffee to be an antioxidant that seems to help in the prevention of colon cancer. Two to four cups daily are optimal.[14] In addition this research revealed the following:

1) The brain functions better when you drink a cup of morning brew—it improves concentration.

2) It boosts stamina before a workout.

3) There is evidence that coffee may help in the prevention of diabetes and Alzheimer's.

4) Coffee reduces the risk of Parkinson's disease and cirrhosis of the liver by eighty percent.

5) Coffee may also lower the risk of Type-2 diabetes and liver cancer.

Surprised? I sure was.

For some coffee may be mildly addictive, but because of its positive properties, it seems a safe bet to drink it daily, especially if you can learn to tolerate it black. Adding cream and/or sugar creates a calorie bomb. If you decide the added sugar and/or cream or milk are worth the calories, go for it. I don't think many of us need extra calories, but there is always the workout factor. It will do the job for you if you don't overload your body with the wrong foods and drinks. I believe under no circumstances should you consume soft drinks for your caffeine boost. There are no benefits to them. Mostly harm.[15] Research suggests they are, at the very least, a contributing factor to the worldwide epidemic of obesity. Thirty percent of the world's population is overweight, which translates to over two billion people.[16] Unfortunately, it appears that this health-destroying tsunami is gradually building.

I take something called probiotics before the evening meal. The human gut contains billions of bacteria, some good and some not so good. Probiotics augment the supply of good food supply.[17] If there's a war going on down there, we need to make sure we have more good-bacteria troops than bad. IBS (Irritable Bowel Syndrome) is very common today, even in younger people. It was never much of an issue for me, but it's not an issue at all since I began taking probiotics. Coincidence? Maybe. Maybe not. I believe they're worth a try.

I never thought I would embrace the idea of vegetable or fruit smoothies. As a Mississippian, that idea was about as foreign to me as a night at the ballet. After all, our main staple, according to some sources, is fried lard. Or fried Twinkies. Whether it moves or doesn't move, you fry it. I love fried chicken and have it now and then. My mom didn't cook that many fresh vegetables. I didn't know there was such a thing as an artichoke when I was a kid. Avocados either. Tomatoes, okra, potatoes, and iceberg lettuce were our main staples.   Carrots? I didn't like them. I didn't like fish either. Or cheese. What was I thinking? I grew up in Biloxi, Mississippi—the Gulf Coast where the seafood was considered some of the best in the world. I was also raised Catholic. What's a Catholic boy to do on meatless Friday when he doesn't like seafood or cheese? I have to tell a tale on myself. One of my most vivid memories was the night I ate seventeen slices of what we called "fried toast." My mom would heat a skillet, throw in several dollops of butter, and lay white bread (Wonder Bread or some such clone) flat in the pan to soak up the butter and brown it slightly. That is fried toast. My Friday go-to meal. Many times, she ended up using a quarter-pound of butter for the toast I consumed. I'm so ashamed . . . but what did I know?

FYI—A short list of natural, healthful foods,[18]

Apples, Bananas, Berries, Melons

Spinach, Kale, Collards, Arugula, Romaine Lettuce, Cucumber

Broccoli

Avocado

Celery

Peppers—bell, red

Cauliflower

Oats

Quinoa

Black Beans

Squashes

Olives and Olive Oil

Coconut

Potatoes

Beets

Artichokes

Asparagus

Mushrooms

Almonds, Cashews, Brazil Nuts

Garlic

Lemons

Chia Seeds

Figs

Sprouts

Root vegetables (radishes, carrots, turnips, rutabaga)

Tomatoes

White Beans

Apple Cider Vinegar

I once was a guy who ate meat every day. Chicken or fish, pork or beef. Had to have it. I thought a meal was not a meal unless it had a hefty portion of meat as the centerpiece. Meat and the amount you believe you need are habits. Habits that can be unhealthy.

As it turns out, I was able to change my habits with the help of an amazing woman, to whom

I've been married for 51 years. My wife is a great cook. One thing she learned from her Chinese acupuncturist is to use meat as a flavoring rather than as a separate large portion to consume. She uses, according to what is available, pork or beef neck bones. She also has used modest amounts of smoked turkey, ham, or lamb in primarily vegetable dishes containing sweet potato, kale, carrots, or any desired vegetable. This makes a soup-like concoction with a strong meat flavor, which for meat lovers is very satisfying, and the soup has moderate but satisfying amounts of meat. I'm a southern boy. I know this sounds like I'm "talkin' trash," but believe me, it's delicious, and I don't miss the big chunk of meat I used to think I couldn't live without.

New evidence suggests that the saturated fat in meat is not the direct cause of heart problems; rather, it's a chemical produced in the gut when meat goes through the digestive process.[19] Could probiotics help with this? No one knows for sure at this time, but I do take them (more on this later). Incidentally, I am not a vegetarian. I eat beef now and then, and I enjoy every bite. But I'm satisfied with one-third of what I used to feel was necessary. I enjoy it even more now than I did back then.

Am I a perfect specimen? Or do I ever stray off the straight and narrow? My wife could write a book listing my falls from grace. But I'll 'fess up. When we take a road trip, we sometimes stop at the "golden arches." Horrors! Well, the coffee there is really good, the best I've run across on the road outside of regular coffee shops. And their Egg McSandwich is not bad, taste wise. Most every time we stop for lunch, I order something called the "buttermilk crispy chicken sandwich." I weakly try to resist but always succumb. Got to have it. But I don't eat like this every day. Of course, these choices may not be for those who need to watch their salt limit or fat consumption. Fast food tends to be high in both.

There are times we, because of convenience or a lack of time, need to buy a food product. Something made by a food conglomerate. I've read dozens of times never to buy anything that has more than five ingredients. If it has more, particularly with a lot of chemical sounding names, avoid it. Or at least minimize your dependency on these processed "food" products. And please try to avoid soft drinks.

I eat chocolate. I've always been a chocoholic. I learned a few years ago that dark chocolate, which is processed from cacao pods grown naturally and harvested from trees in Central and South America, has antioxidant properties, and research has shown the following benefits:[20]

- Lowers cholesterol levels

- Helps prevent cognitive decline

- Reduces the risk of cardiovascular problems

This grade of chocolate also has an effect on mood, along with several other positive properties. I'm not referring to the milk chocolate candy bars you find at the counter at check-out. Healthful chocolate has to have a high percentage of cacao. At this writing, I get an 18-ounce, seventy-two percent cacao bar for $4.99 from Trader Joe's. It's not sweet, but my wife makes candy from it containing raisins or nuts, and it hits me in the chocolate place. Dark chocolate has the advantage of being more satisfying than adulterated versions. It's the real deal.

I am no saint. I eat plenty of foods I wouldn't recommend in this book. I ate far too much sugar when I was younger. Who knew it was one of the worst enemies to our health? The knowledge came later. In study after study, sugar is found to be a contributor to many of our country's health issues. The sugar industry has been brilliant at obfuscation and disinformation that throw into doubt scientific conclusions with strong supporting evidence. But isn't this business as usual? Question any "research" from any organization that is affiliated with the product. At times it is not so obvious. Haven't we all heard that secrets are seldom kept for the right reason?

Regarding sweeteners, there are choices other than sugar or artificial brands. One is stevia, a natural and, at this writing, considered a safe product. Another is a product named Whey Low, which is a low glycemic version of basic sugar. My wife makes a mixture of the two and is satisfied with the resulting taste. Honey is a natural, good sweetener because it has health benefits over and above its function as a sweetener. It is said that if you buy locally harvested honey it can help offset the severity of seasonal allergies. I like it, but it has a unique flavor that can dominate the taste of the beverage or food you want to sweeten.

Water and Other Beverages

When I was a child, I remember hearing this saying: "You can live weeks without food, but only five days without water." I guess that depends on circumstance. If you're in the Gobi Desert, the time frame may alter. The body is mostly made up of water and needs it for the countless and continuous chemical reactions required to sustain a healthy life. Athletic performance deteriorates rapidly—twenty percent or more—when dehydration sets in. It's not a good idea to avoid drinking water, even though I know some people don't care for its taste or absence of taste. When I was younger, I drank plenty of water. My body told me when I was thirsty. But as you age, you lose the ability to feel thirst and need to drink water even when you're not consciously thirsty.[21] I hardly ever feel thirsty now, and if I don't drink, I end up dehydrated. Once I became aware of this while doing the research for this book, I started a new regimen. Several times a day, I pour a tall glass of water (10 ounces or so) and slug it down. I once heard a kidney specialist say that if people drank enough water, he would be out of business.

I've had two kidney stones. Could it be that I've been dehydrated for years? I'm doing what I can, I hope, to avoid a repeat of the stones. They are painful and can be potentially dangerous.

This item may belong under the heading of "Too Much Information," but if you don't know about this, it's something you should know. To find out whether you are well-hydrated or not, check the color of your urine. If it's a pale-yellow color, then you are likely where you need to be. To get more specific about what "pale" means, Google Armstrong Chart. It's like a paint color swatch graph, that will show you the eight different hues of urine and what they mean.

How much water should you drink each day? [22] Some sources say you should drink an ounce of water for every two pounds of body weight. For example, a 144-lb. person should be drinking nine 8-oz. glasses a day. That's a lot. We've all seen people carrying around plastic water bottles. (I'm not a fan of the plastic bottles. They create excess garbage unless recycled, although they do remind you to drink more often. There is also the undesirable BPA factor.) I have a BPA-free, permanent container that I fill with filtered water from Whole Foods. I don't like to drink tap water. Though cities will tell you it's safe, but it has a distinct taste to me, and what does "safe" mean anyway? Research has detected traces of pharmaceuticals and other chemicals that have leached into many of our water systems. For those without access to bulk filtered water, there are several inexpensive filter products on the market to filter your tap water. I have recently started drinking alkaline water, which is also sold at Whole Foods. It costs more, about a buck a gallon versus thirty-nine cents for filtered, but if alkalinity actually inhibits cancer, it could be a good investment.

Water is also necessary for metabolizing fat and alcohol. When we drink alcohol and eat chips or other fatty foods, the body sometimes lacks enough water to work on both, so it decides to metabolize the alcohol first—it's the most detrimental. Without sufficient water to do more, it stores the fat.[23] This usually occurs on the butt and thighs of the ladies and the belly of the men. "Beer belly" may have more truth to it than I once thought. I drink extra glasses of water when I drink alcohol so that it's easier for the body to do its clean-up work. Otherwise, your body will rob water from wherever it can to chemically get rid of alcohol through the liver. Water can even be taken from the large intestine, which can result in constipation. The consequence, particularly if you overdid it, is to become extremely dehydrated. Coffee is a diuretic, making you urinate more than usual. It can be another though lesser problem than alcohol. Bottom line? Drink your water even when you don't feel thirsty.

I do not drink milk—haven't drunk a glass of milk in decades. Occasionally I use some on cereal, but even then, I mostly use almond milk. I didn't like the taste of milk as a child but started drinking it now

117

and then later, believing there were some health benefits. I learned that weight-bearing exercise has more to do with strong bones and that even cows don't drink it after they're weaned. I also take a multivitamin. I learned recently that you should try to get multivitamins without any metals in them—zinc, copper, etc. Reason? There is some suspicion that metals, namely copper, might trigger Alzheimer's Disease.[24] Whether this is true or not, my personal history tells me to exercise caution. Caveat: Multivitamins without metals are not that easy to find.

Wine? Alcohol? Yep. I'm guilty here too. I try to hold myself to 9 or 10 ounces at dinner, but I fail sometimes. Occasionally I'll have a dark beer or two. Maybe a martini. Not all at once because combining is a bad idea. Men can have two drinks a day, women one, according to current research.[25] Some people feel that alcohol is the main reason they've become overweight. It may contribute to weight gain, but for any individual, it's hard to target only one thing as the cause.

In addition to a sufficient amount of water, another ally for weight loss is fiber, a carbohydrate found in nuts, vegetables, fruits, and legumes. It can be either insoluble (nondigestible) or soluble (digestible).[26] It regulates hunger and calorie intake, slowing the system down and making the stomach feel full. Fiber helps our bodies achieve regularity in elimination. Mom used to call it "roughage." Ironically, a peasant diet of vegetable stew with meat flavoring—pork neck bones for example—provides the magic ingredients. One recommended daily fiber estimate for women under fifty is 25 grams daily; for men of the same age, 38 grams.[27] Some of the best sources are apples, pears, strawberries, broccoli, oats, lentils, popcorn, almonds, almost all kinds of beans, avocados, chia seeds, and dark chocolate.[28]

······

FYI—A Green Drink

It's not the green drink. It's a green drink. There are many such recipes to be found in cookbooks and on the Internet. This is just one that I like, and I some-times drink it in the afternoon as a snack. It's a lot better tasting than most of you would think.

2 cups kale or spinach

4 celery stalks

1/2 medium cucumber

1 or 2 tbsp lemon juice

1 tbsp Bragg's Liquid Aminos

1/2 tsp of sriracha or hot sauce (optional)

1/2 cup water or tomato juice or both

Blend till smooth.

······

I've never felt better about what I eat than I do now. Remember a fellow named Jack LaLanne? Some people regarded him as kind of a flake, with his obsession with juicing and wacky-sounding stunts. He was a good promoter. And he lived long and well. He was ninety-six-plus when he went to the Great Juice Bar in the sky. At least in his case, it worked, and I don't see a compelling reason why it shouldn't work for many, maybe even most of us. We all know the common saying, "You are what you eat." Although scholars might disagree about its origin, it came to us long ago and still rings true today.

Most everywhere, people follow the food choices they experienced and enjoyed growing up. Some are very narrow. But there are wonderful choices that, unless you get exposed to them, you can't appreciate them. I was lucky. I got out of the revolving door of one style of food—a basic southern diet—fried meats, potatoes, gravies, and boiled vegetables, using few if any spices—into another universe of different foods prepared in different ways. I made some culinary discoveries that I still love today. It might sound strange, but if you change your diet, your tastes often change as well. What was once your favorite food may not end up being your favorite food. You might still enjoy it, but not to the exclusion of some of the newer tastes you've acquired. That's what makes the human animal such a complex masterpiece. We are enormously adaptable—but only if we give our minds and bodies a chance.

......

When diet is wrong, medicine is of no use. When diet is correct, medicine is of no need. —Ancient Proverb

**Bad choices get you into trouble.
Good choices generally don't.
It takes years to figure out
which is which.**

**If you see food or drink advertised on television, it is probably not anything good for you.
It may be the opposite.**

......

Sidestory

Around 1999, I had the pleasure of working with Dolly Parton on a made-for-TV movie, *Blue Valley Songbird*. (At the time, I thought she might have fashioned herself after Daisy Mae from the *Lil' Abner* comic strip, which ran in many newspapers for forty-three years until 1977.)

I'd had the good fortune of meeting her before, and learned that Dolly is a very intelligent and disciplined lady. She gets up every morning at six a.m. and works until noon writing songs. But as anyone who has worked with her knows, she knows how to have fun. I played her father in a flashback part of the movie. I was kind of a sickie, abusive type. Toward the end of the shooting, she piled the whole cast into a bus and took us to her home in Nashville where she showed us two huge climate-controlled buildings containing memorabilia and costumes from her entire career. The experience was pretty amazing. She provided wine and snacks for the cast. We passed a tennis court on the grounds, and I asked if she played. She said, "No darlin', I don't exercise." When I asked her how she was able to keep her hourglass figure, she answered, "I eat one bite of anything I want."

FYI—By the way, some non-organic foods are considered relatively safe to eat. A partial list follows.[29]

Onions

Avocados

Pineapples

Asparagus

Grapefruit

Mangoes

Kiwis

Mushrooms

Papayas

Sweet Peas

Cantaloupes

Sweet Potatoes

Eggplants

Cabbages

Watermelons

Cauliflowers

The Aging Train: How *You* Can Slow It Down

CHAPTER 9
Sleep and Sex

Good health is a matter of balance between the body, the intellect, and the emotions. If one area is compromised, it will affect the others. If you feel good about yourself, it will show. Well-being will radiate outward toward anyone you meet, and that's how they'll see you. In one of Louise Penny's wonderful Inspector Gamache series mystery books, *Bury Your Dead,* the inspector remarks, "When you have vitality, it's almost impossible to be unattractive."

Sleep

Getting the sleep you need often becomes more difficult as you age. If you exercise and remain active—in other words, have things to do—it tends toward being less of a problem. When folks are sedentary the problem is most acute. Here are some of the recommendations sleep experts suggest.[1]

1) Bed is for sleep. Not reading or watching TV, I-phones, computers or political discussions.

2) Avoid exercise within three hours of bedtime.

3) When you feel sleepy, go to bed. Resist the temptation to stay up because "it's too early." (Sometimes if you miss the "sleepy" window it doesn't come back around for hours.)

4) Try to have a regular schedule as to when you go to bed and when you wake up in the morning.

5) Use melatonin or valerian to regulate sleep cycles if you find either helps.

6) Sex? For some helpful, for others not. (Which I guess means sex should take place earlier in the day, unless opportunity serendipitously intersects with interest—or something like that.)

7) Avoid eating past 6 p.m.

8) Avoid an excess of alcohol – this inhibits sleep. (I have a problem with this one, loving passionately the best thing that ever happened to a grape—wine.)

9) Avoid caffeine late in the day.

10) Avoid naps late in the day

11) Keep your bedroom dark and on the cooler side. It's okay to have a small, plug nightlight to see where you are going when headed to the bathroom

12) Consider using a white-noise machine that helps suppress the various sounds that can interrupt the sleep process. It works for me.

13) If you or your significant other snores, you might try a snoring mouthpiece.

About ten years ago, I bought a device for snoring, and it really helped. There are several on the market from $30-ish to close to $100. It seems pricey to me—everything does to me these days—but if it works, it's worth it. If snoring is a problem, look at the various options online and try one that appeals to you. But if it's your significant other who has the problem, you're on your own.

A crazy positive which happened with a snoring mouthpiece is that when I wear it, it controls my TMJ (temporomandibular joint—the joint that connects the jaw with the skull). The jaw, through time and years of chewing, wears down, and some-times it moves out of place when you sleep. It pops or is very painful when you try to chew food in the morning. It only happens with me in colder weather. I don't know why. I believe when I sleep without the anti-snoring device, the jaw moves into awkward places for long periods of time. The mouthpiece keeps it centered all night.

I don't often have problems with acid reflux, but when I do, I don't take an antacid. I get a glass of cold water and drink it. Water washes down and dilutes the acid, relieving the burn. It also helps to try sleeping on your left side. The stomach has less of an angle to work with, and unless you overeat too late at night or ate something too spicy (or too sugary, which also contributes to acidity), it usually takes care of the problem. If it persists, take a teaspoon of apple cider vinegar and be sure to dilute it in water, at least one eight-ounce glass of water per tablespoon of vinegar. You can also use balsamic vinegar, a gentler dose, which has worked for me. Keep in mind that for some it works, for others, it doesn't. Research results lie on both sides of the fence.[2] It also depends on what is causing the reflux and, as always, chemistry.

Good sleep is as important as just about anything in life. If you're having problems with sleep, give some (or all) of these suggestions a try. Those with severe sleep issues will want to talk to their general practitioners or specialists and possibly take a sleep test.

Sex?

There are those who believe people of a certain age—let's pick an arbitrary number, say sixty-five or older—should be all past that. Au contraire! (The "those" I referred to, may end up changing their belief once they arrive at that "certain age"). Sex, when you're older, doesn't have to be relegated to a scrapbook of fond memories. I was curious and did some research on sex at old-age homes and found that a lot of our more mature citizens are engaging with each other more often than thought.[3] I'll raise a glass to that. There are many good reasons why sex should be part of everyone's life, no matter what age. And it doesn't have to be an all-or-nothing, result-based proposition. Just touching someone and being touched is sometimes a satisfying thing.

The simple act of touching is powerful. Two people who don't touch can drift away from each other so easily. It's a simple way of reconnecting the bond that brought you together in the first place. Take your time. There are a lot of places to stop along the way. It doesn't have to be graded; it doesn't have to result in fireworks. And it doesn't always have to end up with visiting "the golden temple of the Himalayas." (In **Biloxi Blues**—one of Neil Simon's plays—the phrase was used by a young man to indicate a certain female body part.) Sex is whatever you want it to be. It's the mortar that keeps two people connected.

I'm going to make a couple of statements based on personal observation and talking to others regarding the differences between men and women when the subject is sex. Understand that in any behavioral statement, it may or may not apply to you. By the way, ladies, guys do talk, contrary to some opinions I've heard and read. We can and do have deeper conversations when we are sitting around having a few beers—on a golf trip for example, where there is a lot of time that has to be filled, and no women around. Not everyone reading this will agree. This is just my experience. And not everything that guys shared with me may resonate with you, but here goes. For women, whether sex happens or not often depends on mood. For men, mood often depends on whether sex happens or not. For a man—the only gender I can speak for with firsthand knowledge—sex is sometimes as much about alleviating discomfort as it is the pursuit of pleasure. A man who has a physical need is edgy, anxious, and can sometimes be prone to anger. My daughter, who has helped me with this book, asks, "So why DIY?" Some feel it's a viable way to find satisfaction. To me, there is a big difference between physical release and emotional connection as far as the depth of satisfaction goes.

On **Rock Center**, a TV news magazine a few years ago, I happened to see Gabrielle Reece interviewed. She is a world-class volleyball player. She was speaking about her marriage, and she said, in essence, that with both sex and exercise, even if you're not in the mood, you never regret doing them. In my experience, sex and exercise can change mood. It has to do with the rush of endorphins. According to Dr. Oz and other health experts, sex is more than a pleasant diversion; it's healthy for the participants.

I know Cialis and the other erectile drugs are almost prohibitively expensive. But there is an international market that can bypass the ridiculous prices the domestic pharmaceutical companies charge. There are alternatives if you don't want to go outside the U.S. Google the following: Horny Goat Weed (epimedium grandiflorum), aka Rowdy Lamb Herb, Randy Beef Grass, Bishop's Hat (?!), and Ying Yang Huo. It's a leaf that has been found to work much like the pills that big pharma makes obscene profits from. I use it in combination with Ginseng Extract. It works. Not only does it increase nitric oxide to assist blood flow to the right place, but it also seems to do the same for libido. And it's much cheaper. Bonus: it's supposed to work for women. I can't say one way or another about that.

If you want something simpler, you might want to check out Global Pharmacy Plus in Vancouver, B.C.[4] It gives you an alternative source for medications at a fraction of the cost. My experience is that the products are not only cheaper, but they also yield comparable results. As with anything related to unregulated medications, there is always a chance of counterfeiting. In my experience, though, so far, so good.

The Aging Train: How _You_ Can Slow It Down

CHAPTER 10
Supplements

When I began this writing adventure, I decided not to jump into the subject of supplements. I didn't know enough. I also knew it was a subject fraught with all kinds of claims and counterclaims, many of which have proven to be false. The study of supplements is an overgrown jungle of truths, half-truths, and out-and-out lies. Who can you believe? The FDA has chosen to opt-out of the research necessary to prove or disprove the claims. There are far too many supplements to research, and the work is too expensive to do. One compound that was marketed a few years back was glucosamine/chondroitin for joint pain. It claimed to rebuild cartilage, reduce pain, and improve movement. I tried it. It did nothing for me. But that doesn't mean it's not a miracle for everyone else in the world, including you. So back to square one: We are on our own. We each need to take responsibility for our own health-care experience.

With regard to avoiding the subject of supplements, I have since changed my mind a bit. There are good ones that can help and show a significant percentage of effectiveness. I've done some personal research and found what appears to be reliable information, which I will pass along to you. What you decide to take depends on your needs, and if you take prescription medication for any reason, you need to run any supplements by your physician

133

or pharmacist to make sure they don't conflict with your prescribed medications.

When it comes to supplements, my choices, inasmuch as I can know, are tailored specifically for me. If you're unsure of what you need, find a good health-food store and ask for suggestions to tailor your multi to your specific needs, or ask for one that is generally a good mix for your age group and gender. Too many options can be confusing unless there is help available to the consumer. **Consumer Reports** reviewed twenty-one multivitamins.[1] The top two were Kirkland (Costco) and Equate (Walmart). Many others also passed the test of their listed claims. As far as for what you should look for and recommended dosages, WebMD is a good source.[2]

We all know about the alphabet vitamins A, B, C, D, and E. Most of these can be covered with a good multivitamin. Other than the supplements I've mentioned, I take Vitamin C. I don't take Vitamin D. Instead I spend time in the sun. Fifteen minutes a day is all that is needed. I get more sun than some people my age because I play golf, but I religiously use sunscreen. I also wear long-sleeved shirts when outside for an extended time. It seems a waste of sunscreen and time to protect my arms. Why not simply cover them? But I get the requisite fifteen minutes of sunlight on my arms before covering them. I prefer whenever possible to eat the foods that provide vitamins to you naturally. Since there is apparently not much downside to taking daily vitamins, though, I believe it makes good sense to treat a multivitamin like an insurance policy.

Linus Pauling, a lauded biochemist, and two-time Nobel prize winner, was called a quack by his peers for advocating large doses of vitamin C, a powerful antioxidant—1000 mg. daily and sometimes more—to ward off colds, protect against heart disease, and help in cancer therapy.[3] I suggest buying a separate bottle of vitamin C at 500 mg. per capsule or tablet. Take the middle ground, and use 500 mg. in addition to the amount in your multivitamin when you feel a cold coming on.

The Next Level

These are supplements that have targeted uses for certain needs. It's up to us to decide whether they are wise to take, considering our habits or lifestyles. I'll start with the more likely and go toward the more esoteric.

1) Probiotics—Your gut is the home for millions of bacteria, both good and bad. Probiotics provide reinforcements on the good side to keep all the systems healthy. The good guys need to win. A good source is yogurt with live cultures, like lactobacillus acidophilus, for example. Probiotics help with a host of digestive tract problems, and according to *Consumer Reports*, assist with weight loss, lower cholesterol and blood pressure, and improve overall health. I

don't recommend products as a general rule, but **Consumer Reports** has a valuable link for the Top Five Probiotics of 2018.[4] Or talk to your health store experts to tailor your purchases to your needs.

2) Milk thistle—Milk thistle has been called the "Mr. Clean" of the liver,[5] which is the destination for all the toxins in our air and water—the drugs we take, many toxic (listen closely to the drug ads and the side effects)—and the food we eat. Oh, and also the types and amounts of drinks we consume. We're talking adult beverages here. If you do drink alcohol, as I do, (mostly wine of either color, each of which has some good characteristics of its own), milk thistle can protect and enhance your liver function. Moderation is the key. Make sure the extract contains over 70% silymarin. I use a liquid form. Milk thistle has also been used to treat cirrhosis of the liver.

3) CoQ10—Coenzyme Q or Ubiquinol—This is made in the body. It's an antioxidant, and it increases the oxygen available for aerobic exercise. CoQ10 is necessary for the heart to function properly.[6] Research shows that statin drugs tamper with the body's ability to naturally produce this chemical compound.[7] If you take statins, I strongly urge you to consider CoQ10. For further reading on this subject, please see Chapter 3 of OTC Natural Cures.[8]

In addition to improving cardiovascular function, CoQ10 does the same thing for cognitive function, and it combats fatigue and fights off free radicals,[9] truly a jack-of-all-trades supplement.

4) Valerian Root[10] or Melatonin[11] which are natural sleep aids. Pharmaceutical drugs to help you sleep are dangerous for some people.[12] So are OTC concoctions—antihistamines, for example.[13] Read the side effects on the labels. Liver failure, dizziness, forgetfulness, the potential for sleepwalking or hallucinations—the list goes on. Ironically, sleep aids offer, in many cases, poor quality sleep They also offer the possibility of becoming addicted. Try either Valerian or Melatonin (which comes in several strengths) before choosing something that for you may offer more bad than good. (FYI—Valerian root capsules smell somewhere north of awful. But there is no taste, so hold your nose and take it. I usually have no problem going to sleep because one of the necessary ingredients for sleeping well is activity. On those occasions when stress or an overactive brain is keeping me from relaxing and shutting down, I use either valerian root or melatonin. They've both worked.

5) Folic Acid[14]—This B vitamin cuts the risk of heart attacks and strokes. There is a theory that our heart problems are the result of nutrient-deficient food supply. That certainly may

be one factor among a number of possibilities. (Many good multivitamins contain folic acid.)

6) Crushed Garlic Cloves—You must be kidding! No, I'm not. Garlic is an ancient cure for many ailments. The reason I include it here is that one of its great properties is warding off infections. It can shorten the recovery time of colds and other viral illnesses.[15] The cloves can be crushed and eaten, or you can buy it in a pill form from a reputable vitamin shop.

7). Andrographis—One of nature's "antibiotics."[16] When used in conjunction with garlic, it ramps up your immune system and fights against respiratory infections and a host of other infectious invasions. One researcher said the combination of garlic and Andrographis is more effective than astralagus and echinacea, another more common pairing used to fight infection.[17]

8) Saw Palmetto—For prostate health. This is a well-known but controversial supplement for men, used to help with the symptoms of an enlarged prostate.[18] Much of the research says that it is no more effective than a placebo, which frankly surprised me. Like everything else in the drug/supplement world, it depends on who you are listening to and your own experience.

9) Hawthorn—A clot-busting supplement. Helpful in the prevention of several cardiovascular heart conditions, hypertension, and arrhythmia.[19]

10) Aspirin—Some controversy surrounds this common OTC med. It is useful to many on a heart regimen, in small doses, for thinning the blood. As you may know, aspirin can cause gastrointestinal irritation or bleeding.[20] I've never had any problems with it.

11) Omega-3 fatty acid—Found in fish oil and some vegetable sources, this is essential in combating inflammation in the arteries.[21] Inflammation, not cholesterol, is now believed to be the likely culprit in heart disease.[22]

Finally, just because these are mentioned last and aren't as familiar as the above doesn't mean that this category is any less effective or less necessary for some conditions.

1) ALA (alpha-lipoic acid)—A high-level antioxidant that provides first aid for the skin. This supplement can help minimize the wrinkling of old age. In addition, it provides a host of other benefits, ranging from heart and liver health, and exercise-stressed muscles.[23] It also helps with collagen retention and is often called nature's facelift.[24] I hadn't heard of this supplement superstar until I did the research for this section.

2) ALCAR (acetyl-L-Carnitine)—Taken in conjunction with ALA, it provides a powerful combination for both heart and mental health.[25]

••••••

For the purpose of transparency, you should know that I don't take all of these supplements. I do take many of them. I simply wanted to shed light on many of the available useful ones. I try to determine where my individual potential weaknesses and strengths are and match the weaknesses with the correct supplements. Admittedly, it's somewhat of a shot in the dark, but I know my body better than any of my doctors do or anyone else does. I live in it. I know what it's good at and what it's not. We have to be, inasmuch as we can, our own health experts. That way we can communicate with our health professionals on a more realistic level.

And the science of supplements is constantly evolving. I was excited to learn about these newest applications...

The first is stem cell treatment for cartilage replacement, for example, the worn-out meniscus in the knee. Stem cells are taken from another location in the patient and injected into the damaged area. The aim is to regenerate the cartilage, making the knee joint functional and painless again. It has worked for some, but the science is not definitive yet. I ran across a quote that makes sense with regard to trying something like this: "For any treatment to work, the right patient has to walk through the door."

The second is hemp oil. The claims for it are far-reaching—it may help with aches and pains, mood, sleep disorders, digestive problems, diabetes, and the immune system. Time will reveal the best version of the truth. I have a couple of friends who swear by it for stomach issues. I'll be trying it myself soon to see if it can reduce knee pain.

There are many other supplements and herbal resources out there that, considering space and book length, cannot be covered. For example, I have not addressed spices such as ginger and turmeric, which are natural anti-inflammatories.[26] To keep it simple, I've come up with a short list that will help to distill recommendations from varied sources and link common threads among them. Consider taking, at a minimum, the following:

A good multivitamin
Probiotics
CoQ10
Omega 3 fatty acids
Vitamin D3

This is just a starter list. If any other supplements seem to address problems you have, give them a try. If you take other medications, please check with your pharmacist to make sure there are no contraindications. If you want more information, I recommend two books: ***Healthy Aging. A Lifelong Guide to Your Well-being*** by Andrew Weil,[27] a well-known medical doctor who specializes in natural and preventative medicine, and ***Over The Counter Natural Cures, Expanded Edition: Take Charge of Your Health in 30 Days for under $10.***[28] by Shane Ellison, a medicinal chemist.

CHAPTER 11
To Let Someone Operate or Not . . .
That Is the Question

Sooner or later, you will be faced with a decision. Joints—knee and hip for just two—often wear out with time and become compromised and painful in varying degrees. You will have to decide what you need to do—choose to have surgery, or not. As I've mentioned before, I'm not a big fan of medical interventions, as a rule. There are too many variables and agendas(?) when it comes to hospitalization and expensive procedures. Deciding whether an operation is truly needed, can pose a dilemma. Statistics do not always bear out the necessity of "going under the knife." I've looked into it, and the data suggests around 10% to possibly 20% of surgeries are unnecessary.[1] Let's face it, surgeons have no incentive to say "Just stretch and do therapy. You don't need surgery." (There are a few that are honest about non-surgical choices, and bless them.) I will relate my experiences, which won't necessarily apply to you, but may lead you to re-evaluate your options.

Story #1:

About twenty years ago, I had right shoulder pain. Anything done overhead, like throwing a ball or serving a tennis ball, was painful. I went through the orthopedic ritual and had a cortisone shot first.

It felt great for two days and started slowly back down the same painful road. My surgeon said, "You probably have a tear, or it is being irritated (a condition called "impingement") by the acromion bone." This is the bone that fits over the top of the rotator cuff —the series of four muscles that allow the shoulder to have full mobility. X-rays were taken, and he discovered that my acromion was not straight, but bent downward (hooked) on the end and sawed into one of the muscles of the rotator cuff, creating inflammation and the pain I was feeling. This was a congenital problem. Having no better choice, I opted for surgery. The orthopedist was great, and I did my rehab homework religiously. Within weeks, I was hitting a golf ball and playing tennis with no pain. The results couldn't have been better. The surgeon was skilled, saw the problem, and fixed it. He cut off the downward slanted bone and left more room for the cuff to move. I had the same problem show up in my left shoulder a few years later and had the same guy do it. It was a longer rehab because the crooked bone had sawn 60% of the muscle. It took more time to heal, but again the results were great.

Story #2 (a different ending):

A few years ago, I started having knee problems, primarily with the left knee. Sometimes it would hurt like hell, sometimes not at all. It had to do with the meniscus, the cartilage that cushions your knee between the femur and the tibia (upper and lower leg bones). As we age, most of us have some kind of knee issue. It's a joint that takes a lot of punishment and through time ends up frayed or torn, whether you're an athlete or not. But it's an oddball injury. You can have a tear and not feel any pain whatsoever. It can hurt sometimes and not hurt at other times. I'd always heard that a meniscus operation was in many cases ineffective or unnecessary except for the young—those whose bones had not stopped growing. I reluctantly decided to go through the operation, though the older you get, the less likely there will be any benefit. As fate and luck would have it, the surgery had to be canceled. Maybe this was serendipity, because the pain (does it still come and go?) up to now has been manageable, and I can do what I want with minimal problems.

I once talked to an orthopedic PA (physician's assistant) about knee problems, and he told me that runners often come in limping for a consultation. They return a few months later (return why? Post-op? after no procedure?) a follow-up visit, and say there's no pain whatsoever in the problem knee. In my estimation, this is an operation that can be skipped unless you're in pain 24/7 and it's affecting the quality of your life. That's how I approach the entire question of most joint surgery. If the pain is manageable, and you can do pretty much what you want to do, forget the operation. If things become worse, you can always change your mind. Operations are painful, rehab is painful, and unfortunately, you can end up worse off for having done it. Does my knee occasionally hurt? Yep. I believe the cartilage might move out of place—the way a rug sometimes gets lumped up—and that's where the pain comes from. But that's just a layperson's opinion. I ice it, try to put the knee in different positions to see if I can maneuver it back into place, and occasionally use an NSAID—Sodium Naproxen (generic Aleve) is my choice. So far, so good.

Story #3:

At one point my problem was bunions. A bunion is a bony hump on the base of the big toe joint. The big toe, through the years, continues to lean toward the neighboring toe, sometimes going underneath it and displacing it, which can cause pain on the pad of the foot when you walk or run. This can also cause a callus to form on the outside of the big toe. What to do? I knew a few people who had this operation. A surgeon essentially breaks the big toe and shaves the bunion off. Then he or she pins the toe straight and puts it in a boot for three to four months. Painful? Very. No one I spoke with said it was fun. The problem I saw was the three to four months of recovery and no guarantee the bunion would not return. I asked the doctor what else could be done. He said, "Why don't you try taping your second and third toes together?" I did. That was two years ago, and I've had no pain since, and no surgery. The tape pulls the second toe away from the encroaching big toe and stabilizes it. I really appreciated his information. I think I happened on a top ten-percenter on my scale of doctors that do it right. I'm lucky I went to that particular doctor and tried his alternative treatment. And I'm lucky it worked. (I recently saw a news report that the operation has been simplified and recovery is much quicker now.[2] If so, great. But I will tape my toes together until further notice.)

Story #4:

A few years back, I played league tennis for a friend of mine who was out of town. My opponent was a thirty-year-old guy (forty years younger than me—what was I thinking?) who had a huge topspin forehand, somewhat like that of the great tennis player, Rafael Nadal. The ball would hit the court, bite the surface, and leap at me because of its heavy forward rotation. In the first set, he ripped a forehand bomb to my backhand, and I swung late. It hit off-center on my racket and felt as heavy as a shotput. I immediately experienced a sharp, stabbing pain in my right shoulder. I managed to finish the match, but it wasn't fun. I had quite a bit of pain, and it didn't get any better for several days.

Here I was again, going back to the orthopedist. I went through the standard regimen—X-ray, cortisone injection, pain returning—and was predictably told I needed surgery for another torn rotator cuff. No surprise here. This meant several weeks with the arm in a sling, rehab, limited activity, and getting out of shape (it happens quickly when you're older). I made a choice to try physical therapy, not expecting too much, but hoping it might help. The therapy went on for twelve weeks and hurt like hell at first. But after a few treatments, the shoulder started feeling better. The theory is, that although I had a torn muscle, if I strengthened the others sufficiently, they would compensate for the weakness of the damaged muscle. So far, my shoulders are stronger than they have ever been. Every now and then the second shoulder will ache slightly in cold weather, but I can live with that. I play tennis the way I did before, and I avoided the knife. (moving this to conclusion...)

Be mindful—and wary—of NSAIDs (non-steroidal anti-inflammatory drugs). These are the over-the-counter pain remedies like sodium naproxen (Aleve), ibuprofen (Advil, Motrin), and aspirin. Take such drugs sparingly unless the pain is so bad it's ruining your life. Taken to excess, each of those mentioned above can be hard on the stomach, liver, and/or kidneys.[3] I have a brilliant chiropractor friend, who believes that organ damage, primarily the liver, will eventually overtake heart disease as the number one killer. I don't necessarily agree, but it is something to be aware of. Me? I try to take OTC's only occasionally. Maybe once every two weeks (sodium naproxen) when I'm having a bad pain day and I have a tennis match. The rest of the time, I try to avoid them.

One particularly vulnerable area of the body is our back. That said, only under a dire circumstance, like severely reduced mobility, would I even consider a back operation. The spinal cord is a very dangerous area to mess with. One slight mistake, and bad things can happen. I wouldn't consider surgery on my back unless I was suffering and had exhausted every other treatment. Research shows that most back pain can be reduced or eliminated by varying methods: Chiropractic, Yoga, Tai Chi, massage therapy, physical therapy, acupuncture, and biofeedback.[4] In fact, pain of many kinds can be significantly reduced or remediated with prescribed physical therapy, stretching, alternative exercise and OTC treatments. What's more, medical care is constantly evolving. There are some promising new methods to relieve knee pain at the time of this writing.[5]

As for pharmaceutical treatments, opioids are highly addictive and only treat the symptoms. NSAIDs are only partially effective, and they often compromise the user's liver. Surgery is sometimes a fifty-fifty proposition at best. I'm being kind here. I only know of one person who had reasonable results, and he was fairly sedentary. But I've spoken to several friends whose results varied from no difference at all to a need for further surgery.

As you age, we all know there will be pain—neck pain, hip pain, arthritis— pain of all shapes and sizes. How you handle it depends on individual tolerance, how it affects your energy level, and your outlook.

CHAPTER 12
Living Our Best Lives: Time, Energy, Friends, and Laughter

What to do with the time we have?

As we age, we all have to find ways to make life continue to be fun. Life left to its own devices, may not necessarily be fun—it can disintegrate into an endless succession of reality TV, or living in the past—not necessarily anyone's "best life." I believe everyone needs a "lech" - a dear departed friend's non-word, which is short for a lecherous interest, a passion, something that excites you and gets you out of bed in the morning. Hobbies and pastimes give us joy for the time we put into them. Maybe you have a lifelong love of something and can give it more time now or maybe you are looking to re-invent yourself. Take an online personal interest survey, join a "meet-up" group, watch community boards for activity postings. Learning and trying new things keeps us young.

As for me? I continue to write songs, still dreaming of and attempting to catch another "whale" (my word for a song so good, it knocks down all the barriers and becomes a smash hit—a fun fantasy, however unlikely). Writing songs keeps my mind active, along with occasionally trying to solve Sudoku puzzles—which I fail at more often than not. In addition, there is my everyday physical regimen.

Tennis and golf provide playtime. That's the fun stuff for me

This all may sound like too much, and occasionally it is, but I like to juggle a lot of balls. I always have. I've always believed we are all born to be a certain way. There will come a time when I'll have to slow the pace and juggle fewer, but I'll continue to do so until circumstances insist otherwise. You don't have to juggle that many balls. Only the ones you want to. The ones you are passionate about.

I don't want to leave you with the impression that I'm some sort of ego-driven "Iron Man." I constantly assess my energy level and decide what, and how much, I feel I can do. I have found, up to a point, that the more you do, the more you're able to do. And sometimes complete rest is called for. There is nothing etched in stone with regard to a healthy lifestyle. Some days the smartest thing to do is not much. If I have golf scheduled for a certain day, I make sure that I'll have the energy to do it. I never feel guilty when I skip a planned workout or anything else. There is no need to pressure yourself to follow some agenda which may do more harm than good. In any physical regimen, you must follow two rules:

(1) Don't get an injury, and (2) If you are going to make a mistake, make it deciding to do too little rather than too much, which goes back to (1). You can always "catch up" another day. Or not worry about it. By the way, this advice is not intended to build a coalition for the future, to get personal

recognition as some sort of off-the-grid guru. What I'm trying to accomplish is to help you create a dialogue within yourself on what your perceptions are and what your truth will become. That might sound pretentious, but you may take what I say with a grain of salt, or you may take it to heart.

Energy and Time −Spending Them Wisely

We don't get to choose how much time we get in this life, but we can determine how much energy we bring to the time we have. Some days I jump out of bed and for a moment think and feel as though I'm forty. Other days I drag out of bed and feel ninety. That's the way it is. Arthritis is a given for most people who are older, but I have a mission to avoid medications whenever possible. Some people, unfortunately, have disabling pain and can only manage this with the help of medication. I'm fortunate that the pain I have is manageable. As I have made very clear in these pages, I don't like pharmaceuticals because of their side effects. Some people get the benefits advertised, others aren't so lucky. As always it comes down to the infinitesimal but ultimately huge individual differences between every human being. Energy is a finite resource. We have to ask ourselves, what do we want to spend it on and what can we do to replenish it?

Be Wary of what you think you want: Lifestyle and Longevity.

Sometimes we want to pursue a course that conventional wisdom says is unwise. Even dangerous or downright unhealthy. But the desire to "live my life the way I want" is often stronger than the harder but better road. You've seen it with people who smoke. Some can't give it up. They got hooked by the additives tobacco companies originally put into their product -specifically to make sure their customers couldn't quit. And these folks defend their habit full well knowing that it might kill them. It's the same, though in a much subtler way, with food choices. Everything matters. (we do? We eat?) We must recognize that everything we eat, everything we do, affects our energy, and either buys us as much time as possible or else steals time from us. Life demands that we make active choices about what we truly want and then we live with the outcomes of those choices.

Sidestory

There was a fairly well-known and successful country singer I knew who, when we had lunch together, would never get a salad, derisively calling it "rabbit food." To my knowledge, he never ate a salad, or fruit, or many vegetables. He drank a lot of beer and ate meat. He smoked. He ended up having a severe heart attack. He eventually recovered, but then he died a few years after that from lung cancer. Who knows whether his aversion to salads had anything to do with anything? He was a talented singer and not a bad guy, but he unknowingly made bad choices. And paid for them. If he had made better choices, would it have made a difference in his life? We'll never know for sure, but there is at least a reasonable chance it might have.

Friends

Research has been done about how good friends are important to longevity and good times as you go through life.[1] I've always been fortunate to run across people who are special, and, no matter how time or life intervenes, I try to hold on to them and keep in touch with them. If someone is more trouble than he or she is worth—some call this "high maintenance"—don't encourage the friendship. You and your time have value. If you have to jump through too many hoops, it has to be really worth it. If you always feel exhausted or depressed after time with a certain person, chances are that they are not good for you. If spending time with someone leaves you smiling or grateful, that's a good sign. The commitment of friendship requires time and energy, and it must be a two-way street. We all know the demands and rewards of being part of a family and we are born into that network. We don't get a choice in the matter. But we have free will when it comes to friends. Good friends are hard to find so when you're lucky enough to find one, hold on. As you likely know, to have a friend, you have to be a friend. Work to find those special connections and then work to keep them. It will make all the difference as you move through the adventures and the heartaches of aging, to have a support network that has seen you at your best and worst – a group of folks who celebrate the good times and have your back in the tough times.

Pets: The other friends

I believe as we age it's good to have a "critter," as a neighbor calls them. Pets will add a different dimension to your life if you've never had one—whether it be a cat or a dog. As you probably know, a cat is more self-sufficient. Though they are affectionate in their own way, they are more aloof as a species. Dogs are needy, kind of like us guys. They need to be walked or let outside at regular intervals. They don't do litter boxes or put down the toilet seat.

There was a recent study in Sweden that concluded that dog owners were 20% less likely to die of heart disease than the dog-less. Single dog owners had the most striking benefit, a 33% reduced risk compared to their single "no dog" counterparts. Researchers were quick to point out that owning a dog may indicate an overall better lifestyle.[2] If you have the energy and resources to take care of a dog, you are probably healthier in general. But having a dog can make people get moving, taking walks and engaging in other pet-related activities where social interaction is often a part of it. Both physical activity and social interaction are good for us.

You probably can tell by now that I'm a dog guy. As I often say, dogs have been some of the best people I know. They give back more than they ask and don't talk politics. We have had several cats, and there were two really special ones I wish I still had. I must confess the reason I thought they were terrific is that their personalities were a combination of cat and dog behavior—hybrids of sorts. Research shows that petting an animal lowers blood pressure. It's also something to care about other than our aches and pains. Something to love takes us out of ourselves. In the case of dogs, it gets us out of the house, out of our little box and into the sun. Good for vitamin D, and an easy walk is never bad.

If you have a pet, good for you. If not, I'd encourage you to consider one. There's little doubt that cats are easier to take care of in several ways. There are animal shelters with lots of orphan cats and dogs needing a home. With dogs, it's a little more involved. First, if you don't plan to have the dog indoors with you, I would advise you to rethink this. To truly appreciate a dog, he/she has to be a part of the family—even if the "family" is just you. Dogs love human companionship. They thrive on it, and they are incredibly sensitive to your moods. They even come to understand you, with or without words.

I have talked to many owners who adopt "rescue dogs." To a person, they've said, "This was the best dog I ever had." A good rescue organization vets the dogs, so you know it's not likely to be aggressive or too difficult to deal with. Always have a trial period with the dog or cat to see if the fit is right. Be patient. The animals initially don't know what's expected of them. A dog wants to do what you want it to do. No matter how cute, don't make the mistake of getting too large a dog unless you are certain you can handle it. Large dogs can, and sometimes do, walk their owners. And again, be patient. Set up a ritual with your pet. Dogs and children are similar in that they like a routine. Do the same things for and with your dog every day at essentially the same time. Have a place for it to sleep that is their own. You will be rewarded.

Laughter and Attitude

What is the key to longevity? Is it all in the numbers? LDL, HDL, blood pressure, and glucose? Or is it family history? Is it how much or what we eat, or whether or how much we exercise? Some experts have found that, yes, all these things can influence longevity, but the most important thing is attitude.[3] For high stress, impatient individuals or those who can rarely find something to be grateful for—the angry, cynical, curmudgeonly types, the whiners and the complainers about everything under the sun, the gloomers, and doomers—I don't have good news.

You might not live as long as those who find something every day to be thankful for. And if you honestly look long and hard enough, you will find that something. It may be buried under some things you might consider getting rid of. "Cultivate an attitude of gratitude," as a yoga instructor friend says.

Norman Cousins was an American author, an editor of the **Saturday Review** for thirty years, a professor, political journalist, believer in holistic healing, and an undaunted optimist.[4] Returning from a trip to Russia in 1964, he came down with a mysterious illness so debilitating that he had to be hospitalized and wasn't able to get out of bed. His condition slowly continued to deteriorate, and he was told he had little chance of survival. One of his doctors allowed him to leave the hospital and move to a hotel, where he took control of his life, quite literally. He could choose what and when to eat, and instead of dealing with the depressing hospital routine, he had his own regimen—watching Marx Brothers films, taking high doses of vitamin C, keeping a positive attitude, having faith and hope, and laughing at the humorous antics of the Marx Brothers. Though his approach to healing was certainly unorthodox, Cousins said, "I made the joyous discovery that ten minutes of genuine belly laughter had an anesthetic effect and would give me at least two hours of pain-free sleep. When the pain-killing effect of the laughter wore off, we would switch on the motion picture projector again and not infrequently, it would lead to another pain-free interval."

His story was so compelling that in 1984 a TV movie was made—**_Anatomy of an Illness_—dramatizing Mr. Cousins' experience.** There are those in the medical profession who doubt very seriously that laughter cured Mr. Cousins. But something did, and it could have been laughter.

I guess the lesson is, don't forget to laugh. If it's possible, surround yourself with people who have a sense of humor about the world—and themselves. The world will never have a shortage of buffoons (political and otherwise) who can make us laugh, but sometimes we get so stressed, we forget to. Don't get caught in that revolving door, because stress can kill you. Most things are laughable if you allow them to be. I'll quote a dear friend, and wise man, Johnny MacRae, again. When little things didn't go exactly as planned for him, he would say, "That ruined my whole minute." This is something to think about and possibly adopt when those annoying day-to-day things happen that, in the bigger picture of life, really don't matter. It's a choice. "Don't sweat the small stuff," the cliché goes. A lot in life is small stuff when you look at it in the hard light of reason.

One of the things I discovered in researching this book was that quite a few of the legends of comedy have had unusually long lives. Bob Hope and George Burns each lived to be one hundred, Milton Berle, ninety-three, Sid Caesar, ninety-one. Among those still with us at the time of this writing are Carl Reiner, ninety-six, Norman Lear, ninety-six, Mel Brooks, ninety-two, Dick Van Dyke, ninety-three, and the indomitable Betty White at ninety-six.[5] Though any conclusion drawn from how long these comedians have lived would be made purely on anecdotal evidence, I think it is wise to look for laughter wherever you can find it. There just may be something to it. (On those days when you need a good chuckle, google "Steven Wright quotes.")

••••••

"I intend to live forever...
So far, so good."
—Steven Wright, comedian

••••••

CHAPTER 13
A Few More Things Worth Knowing

There are things you may know, and if not you should. I've included a few of them here.

Regarding healthy teeth and gums, I highly recommend flossing every night. It prevents cavities and promotes healthy gums. You only have one set of these. It's wise to take care of them.

FYI— I floss every night before I brush. I have all of my teeth, except for the wisdom teeth that grew in sideways and had to be pulled. When I was younger, I brushed with a regular toothbrush, sawing back and forth. And I didn't floss. Those bad habits started erosion at the gum line—a wearing away of the enamel, creating a ridge that was starting to be sensitive. My dentist told me what was happening, and I started brushing up and down and eventually got an electric toothbrush, which has a circular motion. (No more erosion.) Concerning dentists and X-rays: You know, the every-six-months bite-wings that are part of your regular check-up. I foolishly never questioned this and for forty years allowed this to continue, which was one of the stupidest things I've ever done, health-wise. For forty-plus years, guess what my various dentists found with all those X-rays? Absolutely nothing. But wait, they did find one thing. More money in their pockets.

Consumer Reports recommends far fewer routine X-rays unless something specific is bothering you. Be firm here. Don't allow it. If your dentist insists, find another dentist.

X-rays, if overdone, can be bad for us. Many studies show the wide-ranging potential deleterious effects of X-rays, so, the fewer the better. The reason is that Radiation is cumulative—and builds up over a lifetime. X-Rays do have benefits, such as initial orthopedic evaluation of shoulders, knees, and other bone structures. MRIs are much clearer but more expensive, therefore X-rays are the first test insurance companies will pay for because, though in some cases they prove worthless, they are the least expensive imaging technology.

Regarding the Internet: Again, the 90/10 rule. In my opinion, 90% of Internet content is agenda-driven garbage, to varying degrees. Political propaganda, solicitations, and consumer products all vying for your attention with what is cleverly crafted to pose as truth. Stephen Colbert coined the term "Truthiness," which explains this phenomenon, though he was applying it specifically to politics.

If you are using the world wide web to research and shop, buyer beware especially applies. Unfortunately, wherever money is concerned, the seller's claims might be questionable. As always, you have to do your homework and try to find corroboration from other sources, not the marketers.

Over time I've come to believe that nature pretty much does it right. Our earth is a natural wonder. It can sustain us and keep us healthy if we can keep ourselves from intervening, from "improving" on what is already there. If we've improved on nature yet, I haven't heard about it. The problem is, we can't keep others from trying to do things faster, cheaper, and supposedly better. Mostly they just do them cheaper. All people try to do is create a "product." Something they can sell and own exclusive rights to. It often doesn't matter if it's not effective, or worse yet, harmful. That sounds cynical, but there are many examples to back up what I'm saying despite the exceptions. Wonder drugs that have saved maybe millions of people are in the ten-percent.

We humans are not robots. Robots can be programmed to do or not do certain things. Not us. We will order the seven-layer chocolate cake. The one-too-many glasses of wine. The doughnut. And why not? As long as you get back to your regimen, you can afford a side trip off the straight and narrow every now and then. No guilt allowed. Enjoy your occasional indulgences and do a couple of extra reps in the gym if it makes you feel better.

Diet and exercise are considered two of the main components of good health. But there is a third, perhaps often ignored, component: having fun and as a result leading a longer, happier life. It makes sense to me. What would be the purpose of living a long life if there was no joy, laughter, and just plain fun?

Some of the things we believe are important change with time and knowledge. If you decide to go down a different road, you will experience a different life. The nice thing about changes is that if you don't like the results, you can always go back to what you believe was better. No matter what, don't say you can't. Everyone can to some degree. Don't let your own mind be the mountain you're afraid to climb. Take joy in what you can do, not what you thought you could, but can't. We all have limitations. Try to push—and if possible, go beyond—yours.

••••••

Follow the one who is searching for the truth, not the one who claims he has found it.

—André Gide (and others)

••••••

The Aging Train: How _You_ Can Slow It Down

CHAPTER 14
A Cautionary Tale

I had a completely unexpected wake-up call in 2014. I was on the elliptical trainer at the Green Hills YMCA in Nashville, TN, doing my Tabata. About halfway through, I felt a strange sensation, and almost immediately the lights went out. I had fainted and apparently fallen off the elliptical. When I woke, I was sitting propped up against a wall. Several people were tending to me, one a YMCA worker. He asked if I was dehydrated and whether I had eaten. No to the first, yes to the second. A heart surgeon happened to be working out nearby. When I regained full awareness, he told me I needed a stress test. I was stunned. I said, "I'm in the best shape of my life. How is this possible?" He insisted, saying he would set it up if I needed him to. Wow. I had thought I was bulletproof. Above such nonsense. But I was about to find out I was wrong—almost dead wrong.

I made an appointment with a heart specialist and had two stress tests. The first was negative. The second was inconclusive but, according to an expert interpretation of the data, suspicious. Suspicious enough to go further. The heart specialist, Byron Haitis, then suggested an arteriogram, which would show whether I had any blockage in my arteries. They sedated me for this procedure, and when I woke up, they told me I had a blockage in one of the three heart arteries (left descending coronary artery, for any medical nerds) and though it wasn't serious, they decided to go ahead and place a stent to open the artery. The experience bothered me a lot. I'd thought I was impervious to heart disease. I supposed all the bad, fatty, wonderful southern-fried foods I'd consumed in my early life had come back to haunt me. (Note: I still need a southern-fried chicken fix every now and then.) I was placed on a blood thinner for a while, along with a statin and one baby aspirin a day. I'd always taken a certain pride in not being on any medications, but this was sobering and, frankly, annoying.

After the stent, I was doing fine. Or so I thought. A couple of weeks later, after a workout, I was driving south on Hillsboro Road in Nashville, headed down to our vet's office to pick up some pills for my two dogs. As I approached Harding Road, a busy cross street, I experienced that same weird feeling I'd had on the elliptical trainer. Again like before, the result was almost immediate. Lights out, very little warning. There was no time to pull over and turn the car off or do anything at all. I apparently turned right onto Harding Road, which was not my intention, and hit the rear end of a dump truck parked on neutral ground on the left of the main road. Pure luck prevented me from plowing into one of the several cars waiting for the light to change. There was no damage to speak of to the dump truck, but my car was considered a total loss by the insurance company. The driver, who was quite concerned about me, had been standing outside his truck when the impact occurred and was unharmed. I woke up bleeding from a cut on my chin. I'd worn a seat belt and thankfully had no other injuries. I kept fading in and out of consciousness, kind of in a fog. An ambulance arrived and took me to a local hospital where the medical staff stitched up my chin and asked me questions. They also evaluated me for a concussion, which I didn't have.

Dr. H. then recommended a pacemaker. I didn't hesitate. Apparently, my heart forgot to beat. I have a few athletic friends who have pacemakers for arrhythmias of some sort. Whether there is some connection between arrhythmias and working out all your life, high-intensity work-outs or not, is unknown.

After the procedure, I felt as if I had a pocket watch stuck in my chest. It was set at sixty beats per minute. In other words, it wouldn't let my heart rate drop below this rate. I was told when I blacked out, my heart rate had probably fallen to zero. The brain, not getting enough oxygen, had immediately shut down. I was amazed at the speed of this reaction. After the pacemaker implant, I asked when I could resume my physical activities. Dr. Haitis said that day, right away if I felt up to it. I didn't take him up on that, but he was serious.

As I write this section, it's now been three years since the heart incident, and I'm fine. I do my same workout routine, and, so far, haven't felt any different from the way I felt before the oxygen insufficiency. If I'd been driving on the freeway when the incident happened, I wouldn't be here to write this sentence. Luck is part of the puzzle of living long and well. Some have it, and I did this time. All that to say, sometimes surgery is necessary. Sometimes medicine saves lives. Sometimes we do everything "right" and still come up short. I believe most of us could do a better job of taking time to enjoy the time we have.

Sidestory

A few years ago, somewhere I came across a sweet anecdote about Pablo Casals (1876-1973), the greatest classical cellist of his time and arguably the greatest ever. While in his nineties, he was in a courtyard in Spain practicing when a student walked by and asked, "Master, why are you still practicing?" He answered, quite simply, "Because I think I'm making progress."[2] This to me is the essence of becoming great: maintaining humility and believing you can improve.

To live a full life, we have to embrace the idea of climbing outside the little box we're in, whether we built it or someone else built it for us. The cliché that applies is What's the worst that can happen? The only time limit is mortality. We can make changes at any age.

AFTERWORD

I've always been interested in trying to achieve the best that is within me. Why? Well, why not? Not the best on the national stage or in the Olympic Stadium, but the best as it pertains to the unique individual in all of us. I always felt there is no one else in the race—I'm in a competition with myself. One person is who I am, the other is who I could be. I don't worry about the others in the race. If they have more talent and ability than I do, and if they do the necessary work, they'll "win." My definition of a winner is someone who simply does the work to get better, no matter how great or modest their goals are—I believe that may be the essence of what Oprah means when she says, "living your best life."

As far as we know, we have but one life on this earth. This is not a dress rehearsal, as the saying goes. I've lost people close to me who never learned that personal health is something you have to work at. No one else can do it for you. Health isn't automatic unless you're a genetic marvel. Those are exceedingly rare. Because the human species no longer has to make much effort to acquire food, shelter, and medical treatment, we've been lulled into a false sense of security. The snakes and saber-toothed tigers are now in our food supply, our drug companies, our "health" providers, and our environment. It's either prohibitively expensive or bad politics for government agencies to adequately regulate all the different food products and services that are more harmful than helpful to us. And that, for the most part, leaves our health in our hands.

I have tried to share with friends and family what I've learned by my own experience. I had a copy of Food, Inc., directed by Robert Kenner, an Oscar-nominated documentary about our food supply and how it has been compromised by Big Ag in the name of profit and "convenience." I gave it to many aware and intelligent people, and I was shocked to find out some didn't watch it, one saying sheepishly, "I didn't want to know." To this day, I don't understand that. There are some things our lives depend on we all need to know.

Instead of preaching to you, I'd rather say what I believe. I don't necessarily believe claims regarding food, medicine, or physicians. I buy organic produce, stay healthy enough that I don't have to take medications, and try to find doctors I feel good about. I try to stay out of hospitals unless it's life or death. I believe we can come out of a hospital sicker—or deader—than when you went in. The number of deaths from infections contracted in hospitals is staggering but not widely advertised.[1] Research exists that confirms the proliferation of superbugs (MRSA, for example) related to the indiscriminate use of antibiotics to keep food animals at least alive and gaining weight until they walk their last few steps to packaged hamburger, [2] and to the general overuse of antibiotics in our medical community.

The drugs we used to rely on to fight infections are now toothless because these superbugs have developed immunity.[3]

On exercise, opinions differ. There are those who believe exercise doesn't help with weight loss. I disagree. I believe it depends on what kind of exercise and at what intensity. Those factors were not mentioned by the naysayers. Some did not dispute, however, that exercise has enormous health benefits—the prevention of certain cancers, the lowering of blood pressure, the reduction of cholesterol, improvement with sleep problems and attention span, and an increase in energy and improvement of mood. It's been suggested that exercise might be the world's best natural drug.[4] In the research I've done, I haven't come across any evidence of a pharmaceutical that can compete with the comprehensive benefits of exercise.

I believe that a long life depends on always playing defense. Never forgetting it. I don't walk tightropes I don't have to walk. For me, this means no motorcycles, texting while driving, risky social behavior, using drugs, climbing mountains, going up on ladders after turning seventy, .spelunking, driving drunk, sailing around the world alone in a small boat, riding in helicopters, juggling chainsaws, or handling snakes (even for religious purposes—suggestion: buy a rubber snake.) I'm sure you can think of plenty of others. I'll take chances, but not where death is one of the all-too-present alternatives. Life 101 is dangerous enough. Of course, there are always those who work at dangerous jobs for all kinds of legitimate reasons—firemen, men and women in the military, first responders, roofers, loggers, policemen, and policewomen. Some have a passion for their jobs, some have no choice. Regardless of their reasons, I do appreciate every one of them.

Understand that this book chronicles my journey. Your journey might not look or be anything like mine. And that is as it should be. We are all different, with individual capabilities and needs. I wrote this book to give an account of what I did, what I experienced, and to present some possibilities, not to give anyone hard and fast rules. You get to make your own.

I hope at least some of this gentle essay resonated with you, even if in small ways. Good luck

supply and how it has been compromised by Big Ag in the name of profit and "convenience." I gave it to many aware and intelligent people, and I was shocked to find out some didn't watch it, one saying sheepishly, "I didn't want to know." To this day, I don't understand that. There are some things our lives depend on we all need to know.

Instead of preaching to you, I'd rather say what I believe. I don't necessarily believe claims regarding food, medicine, or physicians. I buy organic produce, stay healthy enough that I don't have to take medications, and try to find doctors I feel good about. I try to stay out of hospitals unless it's life or death. I believe we can come out of a hospital sicker—or deader—than when you went in. The number of deaths from infections contracted in hospitals is staggering but not widely advertised. Research exists that confirms the proliferation of superbugs (MRSA, for example) related to the indiscriminate use of antibiotics to keep food animals at least alive and gaining weight until they walk their last few steps to packaged hamburger, and to the general overuse of antibiotics in our medical community. The drugs we used to rely on to fight infections are now toothless because these superbugs have developed immunity.[4]

On exercise, opinions differ. There are those who believe exercise doesn't help with weight loss. I disagree. I believe it depends on what kind of exercise and at what intensity. Those factors were not mentioned by the naysayers. Some did not dispute, however, that exercise has enormous health benefits—the prevention of certain cancers, the lowering of blood pressure, the reduction of cholesterol, improvement with sleep problems and attention span, and an increase in energy and improvement of mood. It's been suggested that exercise might be the world's best natural drug.[4] In the research I've done, I haven't come across any evidence of a pharmaceutical that can compete with the comprehensive benefits of exercise.

I believe that a long life depends on always playing defense. Never forgetting it. I don't walk tightropes I don't have to walk. For me, this means no motorcycles, texting while driving, risky social behavior, using drugs, climbing mountains, going up on ladders after turning seventy, .spelunking, driving drunk, sailing around the world alone in a small boat, riding in helicopters, juggling chainsaws, or handling snakes (even for religious purposes—suggestion: buy a rubber snake.) I'm sure you can think of plenty of others. I'll take chances, but not where death is one of the all-too-present alternatives. Life 101 is dangerous enough. Of course, there are always those who work at dangerous jobs for all kinds of legitimate reasons—firemen, men and women in the military, first responders, roofers, loggers, policemen and policewomen. Some have a passion for their jobs, some have no choice. Regardless of their reasons, I do appreciate every one of them.

Understand that this book chronicles my journey. Your journey might not look or be anything like mine. And that is as it should be. We are all different, with individual capabilities and needs. I wrote this book to give an account of what I did, what I experienced, and to present some possibilities, not to give anyone hard and fast rules. You get to make your own.

I hope at least some of this gentle essay resonated with you, even if in small ways. Good luck.

••••••

**When it comes to life,
Theodore Geisel got it right...
"Don't cry because it's over; smile
because it happened"**

••••••

A SHORT LIST OF BOOK RECOMMENDATIONS

Over the Counter Natural Cures, Expanded Edition: Take Charge of Your Health in 30 Days with 10 Lifesaving Supplements for Under $10
by Shane Ellison, M.S.

The 4 Hour Body:
An Uncommon Guide to Rapid Fat Loss, Incredible Sex and Becoming Superhuman
by Timothy Ferriss

The Fast Diet:
Lose Weight, Stay Healthy, and Live Longer with the Simple Secret of Intermittent Fasting
by Dr. Michael Mosely and Mimi Spencer

Clean Gut
by Alejandro Junger, M.D.

VB6:
Eat Vegan Before 6:00 to Lose Weight and Restore Your Health . . . for Good
by Mark Bittman

The Blood Sugar Solution:
10-Day Detox Diet
by Mark Hyman, M.D.

It Starts with Food:
Discover the Whole30 and Change Your Life in Unexpected Ways
by Dallas and Melissa Hartwig

Healthy Aging:
A Lifelong Guide to Your Well-Being
by Andrew Weil, M.D.

Secrets of Longevity:
Hundreds of Ways to Live to Be 100
by Dr. Maoshing Ni

The Four Agreements:
A Practical Guide to Personal Freedom
by Don Miguel Ruiz

SOURCES

Chapter 3 Sources
The Big Questions

1) The World Health Organization ranks health and health care for all countries. http://thepatientfactor.com/canadian-health-care-information/world-health-organizations-ranking-of-the-worlds-health-systems/

2) According to Steven Brill in the cover story for *Time* (April 4, 2013), people in the US spend about 20% of GDP on health care. People in other developed countries spend about half of that.

3) Robert Langreth (February 5, 2019) writing in *Bloomberg*, found that people in the US paid an average of $1200 a year for prescription drugs, more than citizens in any other country.

4) Michael Schroeder (September 27, 2016), "Death by Prescription," *US News and World Report*.

5) Because makers of brand-name drugs refused to provide samples of their drugs for development of generic drugs, their drug prices increased by double-digit percentages since 2012 and cost Medicare and Medicaid nearly $12 billion in 2016. Sidney Lupkin (May 23, 2018). "Drugmakers Blamed For Blocking Generics Have Jacked Up Prices And Cost U.S. Billions." *Kaiser Health News*.

6) The U.S. consumer drug advertising boom on television began in 1997, when the FDA relaxed its guidelines relating to broadcast media. Harvard Health

(February, 2017). "Do not get sold on drug advertising." https://www.health.harvard.edu/drugs-and-medications/do-not-get-sold-on-drug-advertising

7) Andrew Weil, M.D. (2007). *Healthy Aging. A Lifelong Guide to Your Well-being*. New York: Penguin.

8) Laura Wagner, (January 4, 2017). "105-year-old cyclist rides 14 miles in an hour en-route to a world record." https://www.npr.org/sections/thetwo-way/2017/01/04/508213332/105-year-old-cyclist-rides-14-miles-in-an-hour-en-route-to-a-world-record

9) Health Prep. "Secrets to aging gracefully." https://healthprep.com/aging/secrets-to-aging-gracefully/?utm_source=google&utm_medium=-search&utm_campaign=1698316511&utm_content=66177941197&utm_term=the%20 aging&gclid=CjwKCAiA_MPuBRB5EiwAHTTvMQhx-foB9AcYYThC5i9bqHXmYyeEnFXRuwm2kV74N-HF_V56pWq4zXxBoC2JEQAvD_BwE

10) Gretchen Reynolds (February 1, 2017). *"How to do the shortest workout possible," New York Times*.

11) Martin Gibala (2017). *The One Minute Workout. Science Shows a Way to Get Fit That's Stronger, Faster, Shorter*. London: Penguin.

Chapter 4 Sources
My Timeline

1) Many scientists considered Linus Pauling a quack for arguing the health benefits of Vitamin C. Some researchers are reconsidering that idea. For example, Hillary Roberts (August 17, 2004) wrote "Vitamin C, Linus Pauling was right all along. A doctor's opinion" in *Medical News Today*

Chapter 5 Sources
Working Out Part 1: Obstacles We Face

1) Chiropractic is a system of therapy focused on the structure of the body, particularly the spine. Chiropractors manipulate the body's alignment to relieve pain and improve function and to help the body heal itself. Harvard Health Publishing (June 6, 2018). "Chiropractic care for pain relief." https://www.health.harvard.edu/pain/chiropractic-care-for-pain-relief

2) Chiropractors do not hold medical degrees, so they aren't medical doctors. They do have extensive training in chiropractic care and are licensed practitioners. *Health Line* (November 1, 2016). https://www.healthline.com/health/are-chiropractors-doctors

3) Neck flexibility is an important factor in driving safety for older adults. Alina Tugend (December 13, 2013) "An alternative to giving up the car keys," *New York Times*

4) Charles Duhigg. (2012). *The Power of Habit*. New York: Random House

Chapter 6 Sources
Overcoming the Obstacles

1) Centers for Disease Control and Prevention (May 11, 2018). "Deaths from falls among persons aged ≥65 years — United States, 2007–2016." https://www.cdc.gov/mmwr/volumes/67/wr/mm6718a1.htm

2) The Mackenzie Institute International. https://www.mckenzieinstitute.org/patients/what-is-the-mckenzie-method/

Chapter 7 Sources
The Secrets to Efficient Exercise-Intensity and Intervals

1) Dean Stattmann & Brittany Smith, "What Tabata is and how it works," *Men's Journal*. https://www.mensjournal.com/health-fitness/tabata-training/

Chapter 8 Sources
Food for Thought_What We Eat and Why I Matters

1) The United States has the greatest number of obese people in the world because of the large population. About 32% of the US population is obese; other countries have higher rates of obesity. http://worldpopulationreview.com/countries/most-obese-countries/

2) Michael Pollan (October 12, 2003). "The way we live now: The (agri)cultural contradictions of obesity," The *New York Times Magazine*. https://michaelpollan.com/articles-archive/the-way-we-live-now-the-agricultural-contradictions-of-obesity/

3) The amount of farmland has remained fairly stable over time, but farms have gotten bigger, and there are fewer family-owned farms. https://www.ers.usda.gov/data-products/ag-and-food-statistics-charting-the-essentials/farming-and-farm-income/

4) A century ago commercial seed banks offered over 300 different seeds for corn. Today only a handful of these are available. https://www.upworthy.com/we-used-to-have-307-kinds-of-corn-guess-how-many-are-left

5) *Consumer Reports* (January 2011). "Ethanol (E85) fuel alternative." https://www.consumerreports.org/cro/2011/01/the-great-ethanol-debate/index.htm

6) Michael Pollan (October 12, 2003). "The way we live now: The (agri)cultural contradictions of obesity," The *New York Times Magazine*. https://michaelpollan.com/articles-archive/the-way-we-live-now-the-agricultural-contradictions-of-obesity/

7) Michael Pollan (October 12, 2003). "The way we live now: The (agri)cultural contradictions of obesity," The *New York Times Magazine* https://michaelpollan.com/articles-archive/the-way-we-live-now-the-agricultural-contradictions-of-obesity/

8) Walton Bello (October 29, 2013). "Twenty-six nations ban GMOs—Why won't the US?" The Nation. https://www.thenation.com/article/twenty-six-countries-ban-gmos-why-wont-us/

9) Crop Trust. "Svalbard global seed vault." https://www.croptrust.org/our-work/svalbard-global-seed-vault/

10) Environmental Working Group. "The dirty dozen." https://organic.org/the-dirty-dozen/

11) Researchers found that mummies showed other diseases of aging, such as brittle bones and hardening of the arteries; this refutes arguments that they did not live long enough to get cancer. https://articles.mercola.com/sites/articles/archive/2010/12/03/cancer-not-found-in-ancient-mummies-appears-to-be-recent-disease.aspx-

12) NBC Nightly News (January 17. 2018) "Time restricted eating can help weight loss, researchers say." https://www.nbcnews.com/health/health-news/time-restricted-eating-can-help-weight-loss-researchers-say-n838486

13) Edison Institute of Nutrition. "15 benefits of drinking lemon water in the morning on an empty stomach."

https://www.edisoninst.com/15-benefits-of-drinking-lemon-water-in-morning-empty-stomach/

14) Kris Gunnars (July 18, 2019). "Coffee and caffeine — How much should you drink?" https://www.healthline.com/nutrition/how-much-coffee-should-you-drink -

15) These beverages are the single largest source of calories and added sugar in the U.S. Researchers have found that higher intake of sugary drinks increases risks for obesity, diabetes, heart disease, gout, and may be associated with earlier death. Harvard School of Public Health. "Sugary drinks," https://www.hsph.harvard.edu/nutritionsource/healthy-drinks/soft-drinks-and-disease/

16) About 2.1 billion people worldwide are overweight or obese. Overweight is defined as Body Mass Index 25 to 29.9. Obesity is defined as Body Mass Index higher that 30. World Population Review. "Most obese countries." http://worldpopulationreview.com/countries/most-obese-countries/

17) Probiotics have been found to aid digestion and improve gut health. Harvard Health (August 22, 2018). "Health benefits of taking probiotics." https://www.health.harvard.edu/vitamins-and-supplements/health-benefits-of-taking-probiotics

   Some foods such as yogurt, sauerkraut, miso soup, soft cheese, sourdough bread, and sour pickles, are also rich in probiotics.

18) Kris Gunnars (June 13, 2019). "50 foods that are super healthy." https://www.healthline.com/nutrition/50-super-healthy-foods

19) James Gallagher (April 8, 2013). "Red meat chemical 'damages heart', say US scientists."

20) Dark chocolate has from 50—90% flavanols, compounds that have been shown to help lower blood pressure and cholesterol, improve cognition and possibly lower the risk of diabetes.
Lisa Drayer (March 8, 2018). "Is dark chocolate healthy?" https://www.cnn.com/2017/10/06/health/dark-chocolate-healthy-food-drayer/index.html

21) John Muir Health. "Dehydration and aging." https://www.johnmuirhealth.com/health-education/health-wellness/senior_health/dehydration-aging.html.

22) Gina Shaw. "Water and your diet: Staying slim and regular with H2O." https://www.webmd.com/diet/features/water-for-weight-loss-diet#1

23) FitDay. "How alcohol affects metabolism." https://www.fitday.com/fitness-articles/fitness/weight-loss/how-alcohol-affects-metabolism.html

24) Emily Main (August 25, 2013). "Is there too much copper In your multivitamin?" https://www.prevention.com/health/memory/a20457994/too-much-copper-in-your-multivitamin/

25) Dietary Guidelines 2015—2020. https://health.gov/dietaryguidelines/2015/guidelines/appendix-9/

26) Soluble fiber, which dissolves in water, can help lower glucose levels as well as help lower blood cholesterol. Foods with soluble fiber include oatmeal, nuts, beans, lentils, apples, and blueberries. Insoluble fiber, which does not dissolve in water, can help food move through your digestive system, promoting regularity and helping prevent constipation. Foods with insoluble fibers include wheat, whole wheat bread, whole grain couscous, brown rice, legumes, carrots, cucumbers, and tomatoes.
The Nutrition Source. Harvard T.H. Chan School of

Public Health. "Fiber." https://www.hsph.harvard.edu/nutritionsource/carbohydrates/fiber/

27) Kathleen M. Zelman. "Fiber: How much do you need?" https://www.webmd.com/diet/guide/fiber-how-much-do-you-need#1

28) Kris Gunnars (August 10, 2018). "22 high-fiber foods you should eat." https://www.healthline.com/nutrition/22-high-fiber-foods

29) August McLaughlin (May 24, 2018). "16 foods you don't always need to buy organic." https://www.livestrong.com/slideshow/1008640-16-foods-dont-always-need-buy-organic/

Chapter 9 Sources
Sleep and Sex

1) National Institute on Aging. "A good night's sleep." https://www.nia.nih.gov/health/good-nights-sleep

2) Andra Picincu & Claudia Thompson (September 13, 2019). "Apple cider benefits for acid reflux." https://www.livestrong.com/article/478034-apple-cider-vinegar-benefits-for-acid-reflux/

3) Marilynn Marchione (August 22, 2007). "Sex and the seniors. Survey shows many elderly people remain frisky." https://www.nytimes.com/2007/08/22/health/22iht-22sex.7216942.html

4) https://www.globalpharmacyplus.com/

Chapter 10 Sources
Supplements

1) *Consumer Reports*. "Choosing the right multivitamin supplement for you. Most we tested were fine, so select by price." https://www.consumerreports.org/cro/2012/05/multivitamins/index.htm

Sources

2) WebMD. "Vitamins and minerals: How much should you take?" https://www.webmd.com/vitamins-and-supplements/vitamins-minerals-how-much-should-you-take#1

3) Dr. Mercola asks, "Was Linus Pauling right about Vitamin C's curative powers after all?" https://articles.mercola.com/sites/articles/archive/2015/11/23/vitamin-c-curative-power.aspx

4) Julia Roe with *Consumer Health Reports* recommends five probiotic supplements. https://consumershealthreport.com/probiotic-supplements/bestprobiotics/

5) Helen West (January 19, 2018) claims there are 7 health benefits of milk thistle. https://www.healthline.com/nutrition/milk-thistle-benefits

6) Arlene Semeco (October 12, 2017) suggests there are several benefits to taking CoQ10. https://www.healthline.com/nutrition/coenzyme-q10

7) Research results are mixed on the impact of taking CoQ10 to counter the effects of statins. Doctors may suggest a trial to see if raising the levels in the blood counters the muscle aches often associated with statin use. CoQ10, however, does reduce the effectiveness of blood thinners. Harvard Health (January, 2015). "4 myths about statins." https://www.health.harvard.edu/heart-health/4-myths-about-statins

8) Shane Ellison (2009). *Over the Counter Natural Cures, Expanded Edition: Take Charge of Your Health in 30 Days with 10 Lifesaving Supplements for under $10*. Napierville: Sourcebooks, Inc.

9) Arlene Semeco (October 12, 2017). 'Health benefits of Q10." https://www.healthline.com/nutrition/coenzyme-q10

10) WebMD. "Valerian." https://www.webmd.com/

vitamins/ai/ingredientmono-870/valerian

11) Lisa Marshall (October 5, 2017) researched the benefits and risks of melatonin for children and adults. "Melatonin benefits, risks: What you need to know." https://www.webmd.com/sleep-disorders/news/20171004/is-natural-sleep-aid-melatonin-safe

12) WebMD. "Understanding the side effects of sleeping pills." https://www.webmd.com/sleep-disorders/guide/understanding-the-side-effects-of-sleeping-pills

13) Andrew Weil (2017). *Mind Over Meds. Know When Drugs Are Necessary, When Alternatives Are Better - and When to Let Your Body Heal on Its Own*. Boston: Little, Brown, and Company.

14) Researchers say a daily dose of folic acid could reduce a person's risk of heart disease and stroke by about 20%. "Folic acid for your heart. Raising your daily dose may help prevent heart disease." https://www.webmd.com/heart-disease/news/20021122/folic-acid-for-your-heart

15) Helen West (March 17, 2016). "How garlic fights colds and the flu." https://www.healthline.com/nutrition/garlic-fights-colds-and-flu

16) Megan Ashton. "The health benefits of andrographis." https://www.livestrong.com/article/414426-the-health-benefits-of-andrographis/

17) Shane Ellison (2009). *Over the Counter Natural Cures, Expanded Edition: Take Charge of Your Health in 30 Days with 10 Lifesaving Supplements for under $10*. Napierville: Sourcebooks, Inc.

18) Shane Ellison (2009). *Over the Counter Natural Cures, Expanded Edition: Take Charge of Your Health in 30 Days with 10 Lifesaving Supplements for under $10*. Napierville: Sourcebooks, Inc.

19) Dr. Mercola (October 24, 2016). "Hawthorn berry for your heart." https://articles.mercola.com/sites/articles/archive/2016/10/24/hawthorn-berry-benefits.aspx

20) The American Heart Association recommended talking to your doctor before taking aspirin for heart disease. http://www.heart.org/en/health-topics/heart-attack/treatment-of-a-heart-attack/aspirin-and-heart-disease

21) Ruari Robertson (December 18, 2018) reported that fish oil may have benefits for health, including heart health. https://www.healthline.com/nutrition/13-benefits-of-fish-oil

22) Johns Hopkins Medicine. "Fight inflammation to help prevent heart disease." https://www.hopkinsmedicine.org/health/wellness-and-prevention/fight-inflammation-to-help-prevent-heart-disease

23) Frieda Wiley (March 14, 2018) reported on the possible health benefits of ALA. https://www.globalhealingcenter.com/natural-health/alpha-lipoic-acid-benefits-side-effects/

24) Shane Ellison (2009). *Over the Counter Natural Cures, Expanded Edition: Take Charge of Your Health in 30 Days with 10 Lifesaving Supplements for under $10.* Napierville: Sourcebooks, Inc.

25) WebMD. "ACETYL-L-CARNITINE," https://www.webmd.com/vitamins/ai/ingredientmono-834/acetyl-l-carnitine

26) Ashley Miller. "What are the health benefits of ginger and turmeric?" https://www.livestrong.com/article/279740-what-are-the-benefits-of-ginger-turmeric/

27) Andrew Weil (2007). *Healthy Aging. A Lifelong Guide to Your Well-being.* New York: Penguin.

28) Ellison, Shane, M.S. *Over the Counter Natural Cures.* Napierville: Sourcebooks, Inc. 2009

Chapter 11 Sources
To Let Someone Operate or Not...That is the Question

1) Researchers suggest that 10–20% of surgeries in some specialties may be unnecessary. Peter Eisler & Barbara Hansen (June 20, 2013). "Doctors perform thousands of unnecessary surgeries," *USA Today.* https://www.usatoday.com/story/news/nation/2013/06/18/unnecessary-surgery-usa-today-investigation/2435009/

2) University Foot and Ankle Institute. "Bunion surgery." https://www.footankleinstitute.com/conditions/bunions/types-of-surgery

3) Harvard Health Publishing. "10 things you should know about common pain relievers." https://www.health.harvard.edu/pain/12-things-you-should-know-about-pain-relievers

4) Karen Mayer Robinson. "Alternative therapies for low back pain." https://www.webmd.com/back-pain/features/alternative-approaches-to-low-back-pain

5) WebMD. "What's new in knee osteoarthritis treatments?" https://www.webmd.com/osteoarthritis/knee-arthritis-treatment-advances#1

Chapter 12 Sources
Living Our Best Lives:
Time, Energy, Friends and Laughter

1) Researchers have found that for people of all ages the absence of social connections carried the same health risk as smoking up to 15 cigarettes a day. Loneliness led to worse outcomes than obesity.

Sources

Emily Sohn (May 26, 2016). "More and more research shows friends are good for your health," *Washington Post*. https://www.washingtonpost.com/national/health-science/more-and-more-research-shows-friends-are-good-for-your-health/2016/05/26/f249e754-204d-11e6-9e7f-57890b612299_story.html?noredirect=on&utm_term=.c064dc21fec5

2) Emily Price (November 20, 2017). "Study finds that dog owners live longer." http://fortune.com/2017/11/20/dog-owners-live-longer/

3) Jane E. Brody (March 27, 2017) reported that positive thinking can be learned by doing some of the following each day:

   - Recognize a positive event each day.
   - Savor that event and log it in a journal or tell someone about it.
   - Start a daily gratitude journal.
   - List a personal strength and note how you used it.
   - Set an attainable goal and note your progress.
   - Report a relatively minor stress and list ways to reappraise the event positively.
   - Recognize and practice small acts of kindness daily.
   - Practice mindfulness, focusing on the here and now rather than the past or future.

   https://www.nytimes.com/2017/03/27/well/live/positive-thinking-may-improve-health-and-extend-life.html

4) Laughter on-Line University. https://www.laugheronlineuniversity.com/norman-cousins-a-laughterpain-case-study/

5) Marlo Thomas (April 26, 2012). "National humor month: Laughing your way to good health." www.huffingtonpost.com/marlo-thomas/national-humor-month_b_1441439.html

Chapter 13 Sources
A Few More Things Worth Knowing

1) *Consumer Reports* (January, 2015). "When to question CT scans and X-rays. Radiation from these tests can increase your cancer risk." https://www.consumerreports.org/cro/2015/01/when-to-skip-ct-scans-and-x-rays/index.htm

2) David Rutherford (July 25, 2018). "The story behind the Bach Cello Suites, and why we still love them today," CPR Classical. https://www.cpr.org/2018/07/25/the-story-behind-the-bach-cello-suites-and-why-we-still-love-them-today/

Afterword

1) Rosemary Black (January 9, 2015). "What your doctor won't tell you about hospital infections." https://www.everydayhealth.com/things-your-doctor-wont-tell-about-hospital-infections/

2) A Greener World. "Human health." https://agreenerworld.org/challenges-and-opportunities/human-health/?gclid=CjwKCAiA_MPuBRB5EiwAHTTvM-cIEMRh8lbTw_Rl_tZH_5XyRDbDPpkO5aXrtOD_1D-DKIphbveXWw4xoCkCwQAvD_BwE

3) Mayo Clinic. "Antibiotics. Are we overusing them?" https://www.mayoclinic.org/healthy-lifestyle/consumer-health/in-depth/antibiotics/art-20045720

4) James Steckelberg. "What are superbugs and what can I do to protect myself from infection?" https://www.mayoclinic.org/diseases-conditions/infectious-diseases/expert-answers/superbugs/faq-20129283